MW01114305

"This is a book that changes lives! Through combining their knowledge and sharing real life situations, Laurie and Dr. George have created a course in Breath Literacy that is easy, effective, and entertaining. Don't miss learning and applying this superpower!"

Peggy Cappy PhD, Master Yoga Teacher,
Creator of *Yoga for the Rest of Us* programs for public television

Praise for *Breath Is Life*

"You have within you an elegant biofeedback device that you have had since the moment you were born and will have for the rest of your life—your breath. *Breath Is Life* is a beautiful blending of art, science and wisdom that can open the key for you to use your breath to ground your body, calm your mind, and deepen your presence. Working with this book may not only help you feel better, it may help you come alive."

> —Henry Emmons MD
> Integrative Psychiatrist with Partners in Resilience
> Author of *The Chemistry of Calm* and *The Chemistry of Joy*

". . . an unusual blending of the neuroscience significance of breath (Breath Literacy) with ancient and contemporary practices that embody breath in action. . . . I love Laurie's sense of humor."

> —Muriel Ryden PhD, RN, FAAN
> Professor Emerita School of Nursing
> University of Minnesota

"The more I read, the more I simply love this book. I see it as one to return to again and again."

> —Francene Hart, Visionary Artist
> Author of *Sacred Geometry of Nature*

"Proper breathing is an overlooked component of athletic performance. *Breath Is Life* demonstrates how breathing and oxygen are essential elements in our quality of life and how working with breath can improve athletic performance."

> —Brian MacLellan
> Two-time NHL Stanley Cup Winner:
> as player for the Calgary Flames, 1989
> as General Manager for the Washington Capitals, 2018

"'Breath Literacy'—the knowledge of how to breathe for heightened personal wellbeing, optimal learning, and academic achievement—is a foundational literacy for all times and for all people.

"The book flows beautifully and I loved every page! The authors share knowledge and wisdom by providing delightful accounts—stories, anecdotes, fables—that bring to light how oxygen exerts a profound impact on all aspects of health—physical, emotional, and psychological.

"Read, Practice, and Transform!"
—Madeleine Hewitt M.Ed
    Executive Director NESA Center
    Near East South Asia Council of Overseas Schools

"Written from the heart . . .
And flows like an effortless, diaphragmatic breath. *Breath Is Life* is a beautiful blend of storytelling, fundamental science, and readily applicable breathing practices. Laurie and George have created an excellent resource that not only shares the infinite power of breath but also provides the tools to experience and embody it."
—Christopher Warden PT, DPT
    Owner / Director
    Merz Integrative Health, Performance, and Physical Therapy

"Thank you, Laurie Ellis-Young and Dr. George Ellis, for writing *Breath Is Life!* Your powerful message is resuscitating humanity's sacred relationship with breath. Ahhhhh."
—Dawn Morningstar
    Founder of Venerable Women LLC
    Master Certified Coach Practitioner
    Author of *Venerable Women: Transform Ourselves, Transform the World*

". . . your expertise comes through on every page . . .
Passion . . . Compassion . . . Fun . . .
You are a treasure trove of powerful information and ways to learn and practice!"
—Debra Magnuson MA, CPCC
    Executive and Career Coach
    Coauthor *Work With Me: A Generational Lens on the New Workforce*

"*Breath Is Life* is a brilliant and persuasive book that emphasizes the value of being truly conscious of how we breathe. It is packed full of good information but also fun and easy to read. The book helped me to remember that good breathing IS good health, and the entire world would benefit by being reminded of that fact. This book will, hopefully, help to manifest that consciousness."

 —Bill Manahan MD
  Assistant Professor Emeritus, Department of Family Medicine
  University of Minnesota, author of *Eat for Health*
  Founder, Minnesota Holistic Medicine Group

"I would highly recommend this book. In 1995 as a student, with Laurie in her "breath" class, I initially was interested in improving my long distance running. Her techniques enhanced my running later in 5 Pikes Peak Marathons, a 100-mile Himalayan, 5-day stage race in the foothills of Mt. Kangchenjunga, India, and another ultra-marathon of 50 miles. Also, I went Himalayan trekking with Laurie and saw the results of her breathing techniques, in every instance."

 —Ron Hagen
  Ironman Athlete and Father

"*Breath Is Life* is not just a book, it's a script for creating a life that is healthy, peaceful, joyful, and fun! This book is an opportunity to explore both the science and the practical application of breath. Learning how to breathe was a critical part of my personal health journey and it was Ms. Laurie who taught me, my staff and the girls in my program, Girls Taking Action, how to use the power of breath to improve our overall health and wellness. Read, practice breathing, and enjoy this journey of discovering and leveraging your breath for a better life!"

 —Dr. Verna Cornelia Price
  The Power of People Leadership Institute
   & The Power of People Consulting Group
  Empowering People of Excellence

"OH MY! What a wonderful book . . . the information is accessible, engaging . . . such a significant contribution and so authentic!"
—Roseanna Gaye Ross PhD
    Professor Emerita in Communication Studies
    St. Cloud State University
    Mediator and Conflict Coach

"The purpose of this marvelous book is to touch and change the quality of daily life, moment by moment, breath by breath, of every reader. Optimal breathing, Laurie and Dr. George observe, is both an art and a science, which also aptly describes their book. It's a book artfully written, filled with inspirational anecdotes and moving vignettes while being totally grounded in scientific research. It's so compelling that not even half way through the preface I was already conscience of my breathing. Being master teachers they use clever acronyms and useful metaphors to help us put to memory practice exercises and key concepts."
—Robert Hetzel PhD
    Former Director of AES
    (American Embassy School)
    New Delhi, India

"*Breath Is Life* is now a key resource on my new self-care journey. Becoming breath literate has enhanced my quality of life. This book is a game changer for anyone who wants to breathe new life into life as you currently know it. I am grateful for being introduced to this vital body of work. Truly—Breath is Life!"
—Annette P. Johnson CPR, MSOL
    The FLY Coach and
    Host of *Living in the Good Space*, YouTube video podcast

"Laurie and Dr. George's book is a celebration of breath as the foundation for greater wellbeing, essential for these chaotic modern times, guiding us toward simple, free techniques for achieving more peace, purpose, and presence.
—Wendlyn A. Stauffer
    Founder, Villa Sumaya Retreat Center
    Lake Atitlán, Guatemala

breath
is life

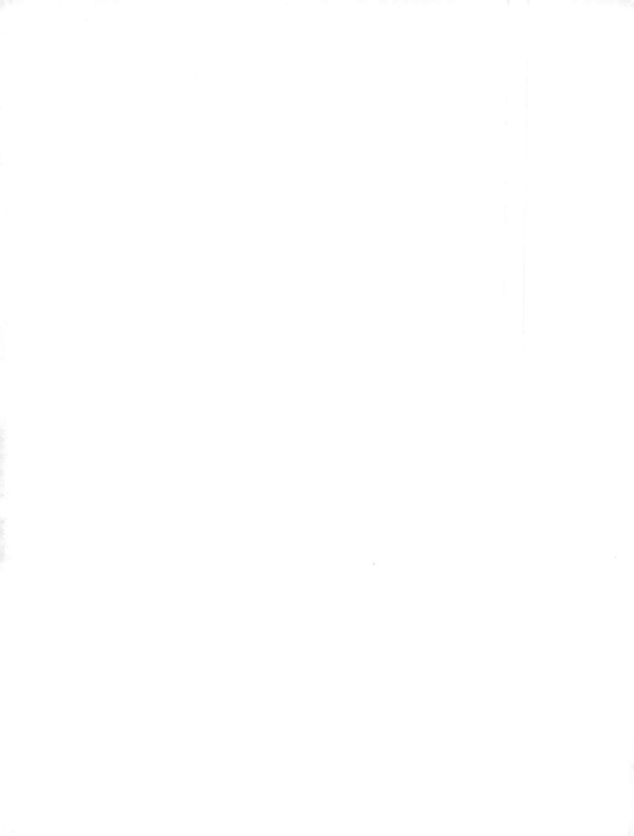

breath
is life

Taking In and Letting Go
How to Live Well, Love Well, BE Well

Laurie Ellis-Young MTC, SYT
with George T. Ellis PsyD

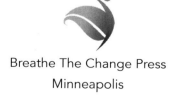

Breathe The Change Press
Minneapolis

Breath Is Life: Taking In and Letting Go, How to Live Well, Love Well, BE Well
Copyright © 2022 Laurie Ellis-Young MTC, SYT and George T. Ellis PsyD, LP.
All rights reserved.

Medical Disclaimer:
The practices that you will learn have many benefits. They are not meant to replace medical attention but to be utilized to aid and enhance any medical treatments.

Published by:
Breathe The Change Press, Minneapolis
Contact: Laurie Ellis-Young
info@BreathLogic.org
breathlogic.org

Front cover design by Kathi Dunn, Dunn+Design.com
Interior design and back cover by Dorie McClelland, springbookdesign.com
Production coordination and photography management by Nancy Chakrin, nancy@nrcgraphics.com
Unless noted otherwise, all photos are by Laurie Ellis-Young
Hot-Air Balloon illustration by Sheryl VanderPol
Polyvagal chart © 2020 Dr. Ruby Jo Walker, rubyjowalker.com, used by permission
Back cover author photo by Jeffrey Hunsberger

ISBN 978-1-7375842-0-9
Cataloging-in-Publication (on request)
First printing, 2022
Printed by Bookmobile in the United States of America

To George

"I add my breath to your breath."

• Pueblo Blessing •

contents

IV your medicine chest

part two: putting understanding into practice

V the right breath at the right time

VI breathing throughout life

foreword

"You must meet Laurie."

I heard this recommendation often when, after fifteen years in family medicine, I began my fellowship in medical anthropology—to study cultures and the health and healing approaches of different communities. This career shift was fueled by the diversity of my patient population and curiosity about the attitudes, beliefs, and healing traditions that helped them make healthcare decisions. At the time I was using basic breathing prompts with my patients, helping guide them during procedures, panic attacks and pain.

"You must meet Laurie."

Who is this woman with such a large global outreach? At our fortuitous meeting I encountered a petite gringita, a dynamo, fluent in Spanish with all the passion and flair of an excellent communicator and in demand speaker. So began our friendship and collaboration over shared languages and a desire to explore the world, and bring back the lessons we learned along the way. We came together from different approaches and studies to form a cross disciplinary, integrative partnership to share the numerous health benefits inherent in breathing.

While serving as a medical consultant for her nonprofit, Breath-Logic, we set up breath training for a hospital health clinic, and wellness programs to help mitigate the effects of job burnout and stress. One clinic program incorporated bilingual training in Diaphragmatic Breathing as part of blood pressure vitals during routine doctor visits. In the process we recognized the benefits of training medical staff in breathing exercises for their own use.

These insights led us to develop specific tools for healthcare workers and for the general public. The "Mindful Medicine 21-day Initiative: Relax, Revitalize, Refocus" was born, a model for stress reduction and life balance that included a Breath Literacy tool kit to use anytime.

From the beginning, Laurie Ellis-Young was ahead of the curve, understanding the connection between well-being and the way we breathe. This awareness allowed her to unleash the power of breath in her own life, and has fueled the work she does to bring this valuable information to others. With Laurie's wonderful sense of humor and abundant knowledge, *Breath Is Life* describes the many ways we can incorporate beneficial breathing techniques into our daily activities. Whether for calming, stress reduction, for focus and energy, to maximize exercise, or for adventures in the Himalayas, this book shares the why, the wow, and the how of working with your breath for optimal well-being.

Breath Is Life is a perfect blend of the beauty and the science of breath. Laurie, together with Dr. George T. Ellis, bring a powerful message about the healing potential of breath to a broad audience. They explain in clear language how to change the way we breathe and the neuroscience behind it. Dr. George helps us discover the beauty of the neurological system and how it can work for or against us, to heal or to hurt, presenting neuroscience lessons in understandable and practical language. Be delighted by the intricacies of the brain, the body and the breath.

I hope every reader will see the urgency and the need to take control of their breathing for better health, become proactive rather than reactive, and move toward preventive medicine. The timing couldn't be any more critical as we experience the challenges of a worldwide pandemic that has left us gasping for breath and reeling, both in mind and body. Step into a master course in Breath Literacy designed to help cultivate a state of calm, healing, and well-being.

"You must meet Laurie!"

Rosa Marroquin MD
Family Medicine

preface

Majestic peaks soared around me in views so spectacular that earlier I'd been moved to tears of gratitude and awe. I felt tears in my eyes again, but these were from exhaustion. At 13,000 feet with 1,000 feet yet to climb before shelter, my body refused to move another step as I struggled to garner stamina.

There on the path to Annapurna Basecamp, the first of several dozen treks in the Himalayas and Andes, I began to realize the way I breathed determined how I moved on a mountain and, more importantly, how I moved through life.

Breath?

Growing up I never gave a thought to my breath. Knowing what I know now, I'm sure my childhood and early life would have been more empowered, healthier, and happier if I had.

Fortunately in my early teens I discovered yoga from a book. I learned to coordinate my breath with movements—a good start, making me at least aware I was breathing and giving me slight glimpses into the gifts of "presence" that breath practice begins to bestow. It was that first trek though in Nepal, that catapulted me to new heights of awareness of breath's potential.

The quest to learn more guided me to many and varied teachers— near and far. I studied qigong, tai chi, meditation, respiratory science, and breathing for healing. I became a Mindfulness-Based Stress Reduction (MBSR) instructor, and first and foremost, I practiced yoga. Originally I thought yoga was only *asanas* (physical postures). I realized soon that it is an actual science of life, of how to attain optimum well-being in life. Essential to this goal is *pranayama*, the yogic science of breath. The yearning to absorb all I could led me around the world to study with amazing teachers and attain varieties of certifications.

My travels were aided by a thirteen-year airline career, which became a training ground to test techniques for coping with high stresses. Not the "high" stresses of a flight crew, rather those of a sedentary reservations agent, and then an always-on-my-feet airport agent. Anyone involved in customer service, phone work, or travel understands. It's both your own and others' stresses—monotony, time concerns, computer problems, unforeseen issues—like the elderly gentleman who flew out of South Africa destined for Aberdeen, Scotland, arriving instead in Aberdeen, South Dakota, thousands of miles out of the way. *What to do?*

First, breathe!

During my years with the airlines, I experienced three problematic mergers. I watched colleagues succumb to stress with nervous breakdowns, eating disorders and other issues. I learned I needed to manage my own nervous system to curtail the stress responses of others. I discovered more layers of the power of breath. Yoga teacher and activist Seane Corn urges, "Breath is everything! Yoga will change your body but the breath will change your life."

At age thirty-six I left the airlines to follow my fervor for yoga and wellness while earning a master's degree in therapeutic counseling emphasizing breath. Nurturing continued passion for travel, I often journeyed alone or took others on expeditions and retreats that tested psycho-physical and spiritual resilience. I witnessed how breath practices empowered each of us in "hairy" situations to keep calm and carry on. From those experiences, my vision crystallized: I became passionate about sharing breath with everyone, not just those interested in trekking, yoga, or meditation. Everyone! No matter one's strength, flexibility, age, gender, race, religion, politics, occupation, or location, we can all benefit immensely from better breathing.

In 2000 I met my life partner George, a psychologist who introduced me to work with humanitarian organizations. In contrast to my discovery of breath awareness and practices through yoga and meditation, George was drawn through research, science, and realizations that implementing this knowledge can change individuals, groups, organizations, and systems. Our paths of time-honored wisdom and modern science converged in the development of Breath Literacy for enhanced health and well-being, physically and psychologically.

As founding director of Breathe The Change, LLC, and cofounder of the nonprofit, BreathLogic, my greatest fulfillment has been witnessing people of so many ages and backgrounds find empowerment and sanctuary inside themselves because of breath. I have taught and presented in wellness and community centers, hospitals, clinics, corporations, schools, universities, and at conferences about arts and healthcare, brain injury, cancer, conflict resolution, education, grief, kindness, leadership, and holistic nursing, among others.

By living and sharing with diverse populations on five continents, George and I have found that people everywhere respond to learning and utilizing the power tools in their breath. Working with one's breath is a profound practice of self-love, and "kindness-inside-out" that helps heal the places deep inside us where we don't feel safe. Breath nourishes, nurtures, and changes us on a cellular level. Of course! Breath is life. So as teacher and author Rieshad Field advises: "Breathe, for God's sake!" The aim of this book is for you to *want* to do just that.

introduction

The single word "Breathe!" is the most concise advice for living. Have you ever looked closely at a loved one and felt a wave of relief when you sensed their breath? Perhaps you've welcomed in new life or held the hand of a loved one as they breathed their last breath—a life gone with an exhalation.

Poignantly, breath signifies life.

For most people, breathing is a routine function performed thousands of times a day with heedless disregard for its amazing potential. Without awareness, your breath is buried treasure. *With awareness, your breath can access unlimited resources to help you flourish in all areas of your life.* Let out a long sigh and feel the promise that statement holds! *Ahhhhhhhhhhhhhhhh!*

In order to show you how, this book is structured as a master course on Breath Literacy with two parts and six sections that focus on the attainment of four main objectives:

1. Understand that how you breathe is both an *art and a science.*
2. Acquire the ability to consciously manage your nervous system.
3. Strengthen a foundation of presence in your body.
   (You may be tempted to hurry past these sections, but please don't! They are essential to your groundwork and "artistry.")
4. Learn how to breathe in the most correct, advantageous ways possible, moment by moment, and in any circumstance.

For readers intrigued by neuroscience, technical information is offered by my husband, Dr. George T. Ellis, a clinical psychologist with specialties in school neuropsychology, trauma, conflict resolution, program development, and Mindfulness-Based Stress Reduction (MBSR).

The practice of conscious breathing is timeless but with the world grappling right now with breathing issues brought on by unprecedented tensions and multiple stresses, knowledge of how to utilize the resources and treasure of our own breath is most timely.

We want you to relish the journey, feeling satisfaction that regarding Breath Literacy you are becoming "an artist and a scientist"—creative and knowledgeable in how you utilize the treasures of breath all throughout your life.

At first reading, this book is meant to help you grasp the richness of breath, then savored as a reference that you can return to over and  over. In order to more easily assimilate knowledge and techniques, chapters end with a symbol of a hot air balloon in the clouds that highlights a summarizing Breathing Essential and a core BLIPP (Breath Literacy's Instant Power Practice) breathing technique. This symbol was chosen to convey the achievement of a higher perspective and ability to soar because of utilization of air, Breath Literacy and BLIPPS.

Try all BLIPPs! Some may resonate with you now, and some may serve as seeds that surface later. They are meant to be integrated with ease, and to be enjoyed. Videos of BLIPP practices and various routines can be found at BreathLogic.org.

You will notice a sprig of eucalyptus leaves gracing many pages. Considered from a sacred tree, eucalyptus leaves were chosen for their beauty and also unique fragrance that entices deeper breathing.

Modern science continues to verify what yogic and Eastern traditions have known for thousands of years. *Our breath is medicinal, and the way we breathe is significant in every area of our lives.* If we breathe better, we sleep better, we have more energy, stronger immune systems, greater focus, and deeper peace.

Dr. George adds:
A foundation for our Breath Literacy course is looking at our nervous systems. The evolution over billions of years from single cell to multicellular life has ultimately resulted in human sentience and the ability to become mindful of our breath. As you read this book, you will learn the importance of breath awareness and breath practices to generate conscious, positive changes in your nervous system and thus your way of being, acting, reacting, and living life.

Welcome . . .

to a journey that can even make a difference in creating a more conscious, peaceful world. That may seem impossible or grandiose, yet master teachers, both East and West, have always advised: "To change the world, you must begin with yourself." And this you can do—one conscious breath at a time. So get comfortable, relax into a full breath, and let's begin.

Breathe, dear Journeyer! Breathe, live long, and prosper!

breath
is life

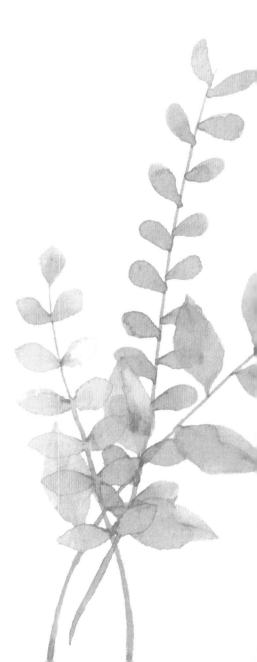

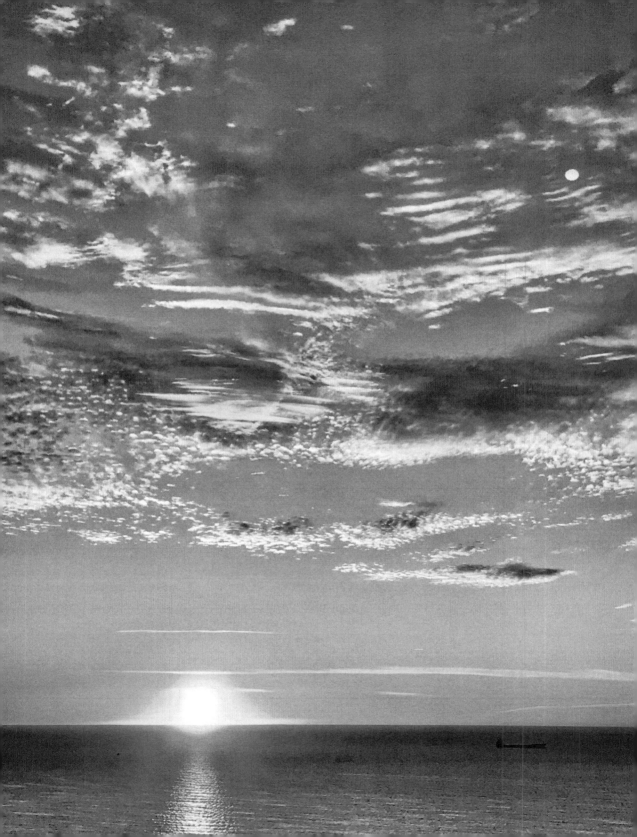

part one

understanding the role
of breathing

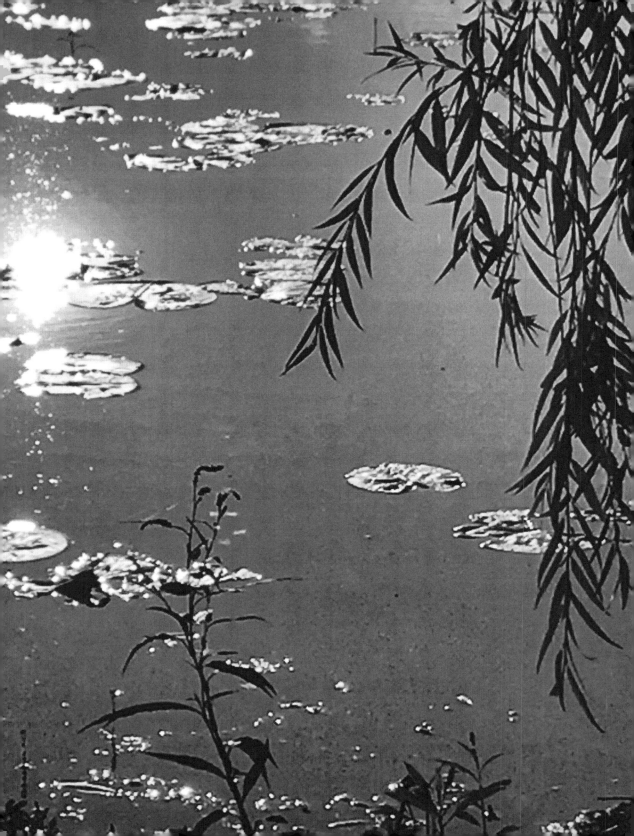

I

why breath?

chapter one

I Breathe, Therefore I Am

Breathing and Being

"I took a deep breath and listened to the old bray of my heart.
I am, I am, I am."
• Sylvia Plath, *The Bell Jar* •

When you wake up in the morning, what do you think about first?
A. A steaming cup of java or tea?
B. What you want to *DO* that day?
C. How you want to *BE / BREATHE* that day?

Most people likely choose both A and B, without C even coming to mind. Our hope is for you to become so captivated with C—how you want to breathe, that A and B will follow naturally. We're not saying "doing" isn't important (or coffee, or tea), but we want to highlight the benefits of *doing* arising out of *being*, and *being* arising out of *breathing*, and what a difference that makes in life. Most of us grow up with messages that who we are does not have anything to do with our breath; who we are comes from what we think, know, and do. These dynamics actually have quite a lot to do with the breath—maybe everything.

Science now reveals that in our busy lives of doing, if we add time for non-doing, we'll become more well-rounded, balanced, healthier, and happier human beings. Yet so often we think, I must be doing something; I must be productive! And actually, that human need and desire is one of the reasons for this book—to show that non-doing is fertile ground for doing. Long ago, Lao Tzu advised, "Search your heart and see the way to do is to be." We can actually be more productive if our doing is rooted in a place of balance and being.

- Our productive lives involve doing,
- Our healthy balance involves being,
- Our being arises out of our breathing!

Genesis 2:7 (NIV) tells us: "Then the Lord God . . . breathed into his nostrils the breath of life; and man became a living being." *The Quran* 15:28–29 (Quranic Arabic Corpus) says: "I . . . have breathed into him of My spirit . . ." From *Big Thunder,* Native American: "The Great Spirit . . . is in the air we breathe." The Hindu *Vedas* are considered "The very breath of God." I could go on.

The course on Breath Literacy in this book demonstrates how adopting techniques of "being" will improve the quality of our lives until our last breath. We will be able to comprehend and appreciate how the ordinary, banal, taken for granted, devalued, underestimated, unappreciated, misunderstood, cast aside, stomped-on (sorry, I'm getting carried away) act of breathing is a most extraordinary and powerful, life-changing tool.

A Fable

The Brain, the Breath, and the Heart go into a bar—a juice bar that is—to discuss which one of them is the most important for a human's health and well-being. The Brain and Heart nod to each other with the assurance that, of course, it has to be between them.

The Brain orders a triple wheat grass (makes its voice deeper), downs it, and thunders, "I AM THE BRAIN! There is no contest! I am the body's control center and I command everything!" Thrusting its arms overhead in a victory position, the Brain roars, "I AM THE MOST IMPORTANT!"

The Heart, mindful of all the plasma it pumps, and loving the color red, orders a tomato/beet juice and sweetly declares, "Oh, Dear Brain, you are magnificent! Truly wonderful, popular, powerful! I just love you!" The Heart demurely sips its drink and rhythmically continues, "But with all due respect, I am the body's center and motor. The Heart gently but courageously affirms, "It is I who am most important!"

Sipping from a glass of oxygen-rich water, the Breath sighs a long, deep, breathy, slow sigh. (The Breath loves to sigh.) *"Ahhhhhhhhhh,* Dear Brain and Dear Heart, you are both remarkable and so significant to the well-being of each and every person, however . . ." Desiring to prove its merit without words, the Breath puts down the water and silently heads out the door.

With the absence of the Breath, soon the Brain can no longer direct, focus, or relegate bodily functions; and the Heart, waning in strength, courage, and compassion, begins to palpitate. Together they panic, gasping with the regretful realization of how for so long they had underestimated the Breath's significance.

"Breath, Breath, please come back!" they beg. "You are vital to everything we do!"

Having anticipated this reaction, the Breath readily returns, beckoning the Brain and Heart to come forward, and whispers (breathily of course), "I'll share a secret. It's not just that I am your fuel and energy source essential for your functioning, how well *I* function determines how well you function."

The Breath humbly sighs, "It is true. *I* am the most important."

"I belong to the beloved, have seen the two worlds as one
and that one call to and know,
first, last, outer, inner,
only that breath breathing human being."
• Rumi "Only Breath" •

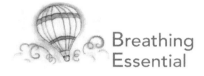

Breathing
Essential

Let awareness of your breath and being
begin the moment you awake.

Practice

Watch your breath. Without changing it,
just notice when you are inhaling,
and when you are exhaling.
Engage this practice throughout your waking hours.

chapter two

BLIPPS

Breath Literacy's Instant Power Practices

Blip . . . blip . . . blip . . .

While sitting in the ICU hospital room, the machine connected to the patient seemed to strive to communicate. Was I imagining this or were those blips trying to ask: "Between the first breath and the last—what does it all really mean?" How many *blips*—moments of our lives—do we live with presence and intention? How many are just a series of robot-like blips of mindlessness and busyness?

Busyness is a factor of modern life, and whether you're over-whelmed with busyness or feel it's under control, it merits a look. Social activist and author Thomas Merton wrote: "To allow oneself to be carried away by a multitude of conflicting concerns, to surrender to too many demands, to commit oneself to too many projects, to want to help everyone in everything, is to succumb to violence."

Busyness as a form of violence may sound like extreme exaggeration, but I ask you to ponder this for a moment. Busyness certainly is not usually a form of conscious aggression; nevertheless, there can be "busyness=violence" repercussions created by society's ingrained expectations that compel over-scheduling, overachieving, and societal pressures to be Superwoman, Superman, Super-teen/child/parent/grandparent. The pressure is on! Busyness can contribute to demanding overactivity, or conversely, arduous underactivity—getting a lot done but being sedentary while we do it (like computer work). This can mean not enough exercise, stiff joints, poor posture, and not breathing well, resulting in poor digestion, poor sleep, and other issues.

Conscious busyness is one thing, but unconscious busyness can end up becoming a vicious and vacuous cycle. Besides not being kind or caring to ourselves, we can end up being unkind to others, negative and reactive, with a predisposition to lashing out. Before you know it, there's contention, clash, and conflict, leading to arguments, fights, and behaviors we're sorry for later. Sometimes it takes having ourselves or someone we love hooked up to one of those machines that breathes for us, before we slow down to pay attention to what we really realize is important.

Blip . . . blip . . . blip . . .

How we are breathing is a barometer for how we are living. In our busy, often-chaotic lives, we can lose the essence of who we are. We become *human-doings*, and *human-goings*, and now in this age of information and accelerated technology, *human-knowings*. With this added identity, it's more essential than ever to balance the searching outside ourselves, and the internet, with exploring our *inner*net.

Masters tell us that peace, happiness, and balance are "inside jobs." Finding the perfect data or bargain may make us happy short term, but programming moments to pause, drop inside, and nurture ourselves as *human BEings* will add up to greater, long-term happiness and health.

Often when we pause to notice our breath, we may find we're actually not breathing. Other times, with life feeling harried, hard, and hectic, we may find our breath seeming to race a mile a minute. *What to do?* How can we change or manage this craziness?

Sitting for hours in hospital rooms with "*blip* machines" barely keeping my loved ones alive made me think a lot about life, death, breath, and those *blips*—as moment-by-moment ways we experience life. As I love words, alliteration, and acronyms, I began to entertain myself pondering different types of *blips*:

b busily /barely /blunderingly

l languishing /lamenting /lingering

i in

p pain /panic /paranoia /pessimism /pandemonium

We've all experienced those types of *blips* sometime or other—hopefully not for too long without at least some respite. I also reflected on other *blips*:

b bountifully /blessedly /blissfully

l living /loving /laughing

i in

p purpose /peace /passion /playfulness /pause

Later, when I again pondered the sound and significance of blips—I had one of those "Ah ha!" moments. I asked myself, "So how do we turn the blips of just surviving into thoroughly thriving?"

That question became the key to what this book is about: living a life of engaging conscious, intentional, positive *blips*—the capitalized BLIPP of: *Breath Literacy's Instant Power Practices*—utilizing our breath purposely for presence, peace, empowerment, health, connections, and greatest well-being.

BLIPPs is the name we give to the tools and techniques we share throughout this book. For short, think of a BLIPP as an Instant Power Practice. You can apply a BLIPP in a *blip* of time, anywhere, any moment. For example, the practice of pausing to know whether you are inhaling or exhaling is a BLIPP. You can insert this practice into practically any conversation, pastime, task, movement, or activity. By integrating BLIPPs into our daily lives, we can accomplish, create, and produce in a manner that is more kind to ourselves, balanced, conscious, and peaceful. We can begin to shift from breathing to survive to breathing to thrive.

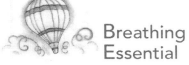

Breathing Essential

How we are breathing is how we are living.

BLIPP

Find ways to pay attention to a full inhalation and exhalation at least once each waking hour for the entire day.
Feel the power of these moments.

chapter three

What Nerve!

Our Nervous System

"Oh, the nerves, the nerves;
the mysteries of this machine called man."
• Charles Dickens •

Tremendous advances in neuroscience have occurred in the last two decades and in these unparalleled times that we are in, neuroscience has gone from being the domain of scientists and doctors to being discussed and implemented by educators, parents, mental health professionals, and others interested in mindfulness and breath.

Dr. George adds:

As a foundation for Breath Literacy, let's look at our human nervous system. For most of us, this is a daunting subject. When the term neuroscience is mentioned, some peoples' eyes glaze over, or they want to "run for the hills." I request that you lend me your trust as we meander together through this interesting "forest of information."

I will only point out what is absolutely necessary for appreciating what your breath practices will actually accomplish on physiological and psychological levels.

Okay, take in a deep breath, let go, *"Ahhhhhhhhh,"* and let's go forest diving. The human nervous system is the most organized and complex system in the human body. Our nervous system receives and interprets information from our senses and transmits impulses to our brain. Our brain uses the information it receives to coordinate all of our actions, reactions, thoughts, emotions, and behaviors.

As you read this book, you will learn the importance of breath awareness and breath practices to generate conscious positive changes in your nervous system and thus your way of being, acting, reacting, and living life.

Imagine that you are at a large party with music, food, drinks, people bumping into each other, laughter, and conversations. Noise, smells, tastes, temperature, eye contact, gestures, facial expressions of all types, people you want to see, those you'd rather not see, and expectations from yourself and others regarding how you should interact, respond, and be, are all assailing you simultaneously. Now amidst this tumult, take a moment to breathe a gentle full breath and allow all the clamor to recede from consciousness.

You are essentially at a sensory party (large or small) every second of your waking life. As you read this paragraph, you are experiencing sensory stimulation from all areas your body touches (clothing, chair, floor, book), temperature, sound, vision, and smell. Luckily, we are not aware of most of this incoming information and inundating bits of data. If we were, we'd likely be profoundly over-whelmed and feel like we were going crazy.

The human nervous system takes all of this sensory information and, mostly beyond our conscious awareness, processes, inte-grates, and coordinates it, unless it reaches a level where our brain makes us pay attention. For example, a hot stove, bees buzzing around the ears, a car honking, the smell of fire, or discomfort from sitting too long.

Our nervous system is made up of the *central nervous system (CNS)* and the *peripheral nervous system (PNS)*. The CNS consists of the brain and the spinal cord, and the PNS consists of everything outside the CNS.

Through our senses, the PNS sends thousands of inputs happening around us to the CNS, which organizes, makes sense of it, and then coordinates the body's responses.

The Peripheral Nervous System (PNS)

The PNS is called peripheral because it is outside the CNS, sending information back and forth to the CNS via bundles of nerve fibers (neurons). The PNS is divided into the somatic and the autonomic nervous system.

The Somatic Sensory System

sends inputs for the skin (temperature, pain, touch), eyes (colors, shapes), and ears (decibels, pitch, tone) to the CNS. Also receiving instructions / data from the CNS, it will respond, for example, by contracting or relaxing muscles.

The Autonomic Nervous System (ANS)

is subdivided into the sympathetic—the "fight or flight" system, and the parasympathetic—the "rest and digest" system. These branches are a major focus in this book and will be addressed often.

Optimal health results when all parts are working well, like impeccably choreographed dancers or sports teams that have played together long enough to be in perfect sync. A major point is that diligently integrating the breathwork taught in these pages will maximize healthy functioning of the entire nervous system and thereby optimize physical, emotional, and mental health. If this seems a little overwhelming, hang in there, it will all come together.

Triune Brain—Paul D. MacLean

In the 1960s, neuroscientist Paul MacLean indicated that the human brain is organized hierarchically based on our evolutionary roots, and has three regions.

1. reptilian or primal brain=the most ancient and the foundation of the brain
2. mammalian or emotional brain=limbic system
3. neo-mammalian or rational brain=neocortex

Unlike computer programs that are deleted and replaced by new programs and software, the human brain, evolving over millions of years, has grown to meet new challenges by preserving the old as well as developing new regions.

Neurons

Our ability to think, analyze, interpret, move, and perform most functions is due to brain cells. The human nervous system contains about 1.1 trillion cells; about 10 percent (100 billion) are specialized cells called neurons; of which there are about 150 different types. The rest of approximately one trillion cells are called glial cells. Without these 100 billion neurons, we would not be able to function, and without the underappreciated glial cells, neurons would not be able to function. (Imagine neurons like big movie stars, and glial cells as the supporting cast and crew.)

Neurons have gained fame because of neuroplasticity, the brain's ability to change, to create and delete neural pathways, something science only recently substantiated. This neural organization and reorganization occur all of the time; the essential question is, can we direct this reorganization in a manner that supports how we want to be and live in the world? The answer: Yes!

The Central Nervous System (CNS)

A few years ago, I had the opportunity to dissect a human brain. Holding this small firm organ smelling of formaldehyde, I found it hard not to think of its former owner: what were his or her dreams, hopes, fears, and loves? This person donated their brain to science for someone to study and learn. I felt grateful.

The brain is divided into two halves, a left and a right hemisphere, which communicate with each other through neurons. Each hemisphere controls the opposite side of the body.

Hemispheres

Over the years, there has been significant misunderstanding regarding the hemisphere's roles and functions. In *The Master, and His Emissary* (2009), an exhaustive review of research on the divided brain, author, phychiatrist Iain McGilchrist reports that both hemispheres fire with and manage everything we hear, think, say, do, and feel. In other words, both hemispheres are activated almost always for everything we experience.

The issue is not *what* each hemisphere does, but *how* each one approaches these tasks, an important distinction because both deal with language, visuospatial tasks, perceptions, emotions, and behavior. Essentially, each hemisphere looks through a different set of glasses. Metaphorically speaking, there are two of you in one body with "each of you" viewing your world through dissimilar lenses and approaching the same task from different perspectives. In order to experience the fullness of who we are, we need input from both hemispheres.

The brain can be conceptualized as having a forebrain, midbrain, and hindbrain. The forebrain, the home of reason, sensory processing, and motor movement, can be divided into four lobes that communicate with each other in various ways:

Frontal lobe: The seat of voluntary movement, parts of speech, and cognition (thinking), planning, reasoning, and problem solving.

Parietal lobe: Processes and integrates sensory information such as touch, temperature, taste, and movement.

Temporal lobe: Associated with perception, hearing, memory, and parts of speech.

Occipital lobe: Processes vision.

The *autonomic nervous system (ANS)* plays an essential role in keeping the body's internal environment in proper balance—homeostasis. Imagine if you consciously needed to maintain your blood sugar levels, regulate your body temperature, and evaluate carbon dioxide levels in your blood and breathe. Luckily the ANS does this for us. In subsequent chapters, we discuss how the ANS sympathetic and parasympathetic systems function and relate to our breath in regards to stress, interpersonal relationships, and our psycho-physical well-being.

As a final point, the only aspect of the ANS, or any system in the body under voluntary control, is our breath. Thus our breath can become a bridge between our body and mind to consciously change our psychological, emotional, and physiological states. *The breath is both a part of our nervous system and a means to transform it. In other words, our breath can change our brains.*

Do you realize the implications?
Ahhhhhhhhhhhhhh!

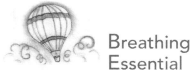

Breathing Essential

Your breath can both excite or calm your nerves.

BLIPP

Become aware of your breath without changing it.
Just notice how watching your breath makes you feel.

chapter four

Magic in the Air

Oxygen as Nourishment

Thank goodness we don't have to remember to breathe. If we did, it would be a constant "Oh no, another one down!" Nevertheless, we hope to inspire you to want to *remember* to breathe and consciously harness the power that is fueled by oxygen—our lifeblood. For homeostasis and optimal well-being, our brains require immense amounts of oxygen. Without this "magic in the air," the multitudes of miraculous, multifarious, *maaahhhhhvelous*, fabulous, far-out functions our brains perform could not take place. (I do love alliteration for emphasis!)

I first experienced the significance of oxygen at age twenty-five when I flew into La Paz, Bolivia, at 13,650 ft. I'd been warned about *soroche* (altitude sickness), but my friend Suzie and I felt impervious. So excited to explore, after hastily dropping our packs at the hotel, we practically sprinted up a long, steep hill. I should say, we started to sprint. Within minutes, it felt like the heavens opened and an axe came down, slicing open our heads. We could barely limp back to our hotel to lay supine in total stillness to give our bodies a chance to assimilate.

We were felled and humbled. Striving to remain motionless, I almost wanted to die. My eyeballs and even my eyelashes ached. All I could do to deal with the pain was *be* with my breath. A great gift in this experience is that later, when I began to trek in the high Himalayas and Andes, I had already acquired healthy respect for the body's need to acclimate to an environment with far less oxygen. I would not let that happen again.

In *The Complete Breath*, Jim Morningstar points out, "There is an expanding recognition that the source of much illness and disease is a lack of oxygenation."

Oxygen is the prime detoxifier of the human body; around 70 percent of all toxins leave the body through the breath. Oxygen "feeds" us—our cells and our brains—whether we notice that or not, which is one of the reasons we usually take it for granted unless, of course, we are gasping for air. Then we put it at the top of our gratitude list.

Dr. George adds:

Two essential points to remember about oxygen, "the magic in our air":

1. Oxygen is essential for all of our brain's functions.
2. The act of breathing is our brain's main supplier of oxygen.

Our brain weighs about 2 percent of our body weight and is fueled by oxygen and glucose. At rest, this amazing organ utilizes about 20 percent of our body's total circulating oxygen and much more during exercise. Oxygen fuels our brain cells. How we breathe dictates how much oxygen is present to our brain, impacting all aspects of functioning (thinking, attitude, feelings, and actions).

For example, shallow chest breathing, something many people with depression and anxiety experience, not only limits the amount of oxygen our bodies and brains receive, it is likely a manifestation of our emotional state. I've worked with many people who faced anxiety and depression, and as their breathing deepened, lengthened, and slowed, many experienced changes in their attitudes and emotional states. Now breath was not the only variable involved in their changes, but my clients and I believed that it had a major positive influence.

Our bodies utilize three main fuels: food, water, and oxygen. We can live weeks without food, days without water, but only minutes without oxygen. The single most-important substance taken into the body, oxygen is essential in every chemical reaction important to human physiology.

- Oxygen aids our cells in metabolizing nutrients for energy, maintenance, repair, and healing.
- What occurs in a heart attack is the ultimate deprivation of oxygen.
- Lack of oxygen is a factor in immune-depressive illnesses.
- Breathing is our chief body cleanser; oxygen aids the elimination of wastes, debris, toxins, and body pollution.
- Oxygen helps burn fat.
- The ways we intake oxygen and release carbon dioxide have a direct effect on every organ, gland, and system in the body.
- Oxygen is the most essential factor for adenosine triphosphate (ATP), the chemical basis of energy production in our bodies.
- Inadequate oxygen results in lowered vitality, disease, and premature aging.

After several hiking journeys in Nepal, my friend Kathy and I decided we were ready for the higher altitude of Mt. Everest Basecamp. We flew into Lukla, the closest airport, deplaning into unexpected excitement and an eager crowd of locals, trekkers, and Tibetan monks clad in red robes. A huge fortieth-year anniversary banner welcomed Sir Edmund Hillary and members of the first expedition to reach the summit. Anticipation was palpable. Hillary had become a hero for the Nepalese and they sang his praises. Enamored with this country and its people, he continually returned to set up schools, humanitarian programs, and environmental projects.

Within half an hour a whirling helicopter landed, and the esteemed mountaineer stepped down into the admiring masses. Hillary has talked often about the significance of oxygen.

> "It was 11:30 a.m. My first sensation was one of relief—
> relief that the long grind was over, that the summit
> had been reached before our oxygen supplies
> had dropped to a critical level;
> and relief that in the end the mountain
> had been kind to us. . . ."
>
> •   Sir Edmund Hillary   •

Everest was the first route I'd taken where trekkers were advised to sleep two nights in the same place in order to acclimate to lower oxygen levels before climbing higher. On the second day at snow-covered Pheriche, 16,340 feet, I went out hiking with Hari, our porter / guide. We watched a man, Brett, sprinting up a steep, white incline. I immediately recalled my painful experience trying to run up a hill in Bolivia. And we were 2,000 feet higher than that hill!

Very concerned, Hari called out to him, expressing that rushing in that altitude was dangerous. "*Dhai* (older brother), wait!"

"No problem," Brett arrogantly dismissed Hari as he dashed away, "I'm from Colorado and the Rockies."

Hari worriedly shook his head and said, "He no be Rockies. He be Himalaya. He be sorry!"

Pheriche now has emergency oxygen provisions, but then they did not. That evening at the teahouse, we heard someone had acute mountain sickness (AMS): symptoms resembling a horrific hangover, carbon monoxide poisoning, and the flu. The next morning, at first light, we saw it was the "Colorado Kid." Looking like death warmed over, he'd spent the entire night in intense pain, unpleasantly involving vomit and diarrhea. His eyes were crossed, and helpers on either side supported him from collapsing. As they prepared to descend, Brett's dream of reaching Mount Everest evaporated into thin air. At least below he'd have more oxygen, his condition's only cure.

With compassion, Hari wished him well. For Kathy and me, the continued hike to over 18,000 feet demonstrated to us the necessity of oxygen for anything we wanted to do—be it think, sleep, or move.

It's important to know that the effects of oxygen deprivation can be experienced even at low altitudes. People at sea level, breathing short, shallow upper chest breaths experience the same type of oxygen deficiency that can occur in high mountains. Usually not full-scale AMS but repressed immune systems can cause low-grade anxiety, weakness, depression, and inability to focus. To make matters worse, the resulting imbalanced metabolism and consequential hyper-activity or lethargy can cause mild or excessive weight loss or weight gain. According to Edward McCabe MD, "Viruses and microbes live best in low-oxygen environments. They are anaerobic. That means: raise the oxygen environment around them and they die."In life, oxygen is necessary for "peak" performance.

Whether to physically climb a mountain or metaphorically feel physically, emotionally, intellectually, personally, or professionally "at the top," oxygen can make the difference. Doesn't this make you want to breathe better?

We've only just begun!

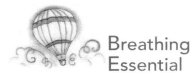

Breathing
Essential

Think of your breathing and oxygen as essential elements in how you live your life.

BLIPP

Watch your breath. Without changing it, notice when you are inhaling, and notice when you are exhaling. Notice the flow from one into the other.

chapter five

Your Brain and Your *"Inner*net"

Shallow Breathing and Feeling Safe

Are you or others you know and love . . .

- living sedentary lifestyles because of work or other circumstances?
- physically incapacitated for any reason? In a wheelchair, bed-ridden, moving slowly about with a cast, crutches, or walker?
- dealing with grief and profound heartache?
- anxious, depressed, overly stressed, sleep deprived, or sleep inundated?

If you see yourself or others here, chances are you all have something in common—not breathing effectively. To put it mildly, this is not "hunky dory."

I often begin workshops with the question, "Why are you here?" Many participants, either hesitantly disclose or adamantly admit, one after another, "I am a shallow breather." These frequent responses prompted me to imagine forming a twelve-step Shallow Breathers Anonymous (SBA) organization. The truth is, unless we practice deepening our breathing, we'd all be members.

Shallow breathing can be like "giving the finger" to life. Now I don't mean this in the same way as someone experiencing road rage. It's meant more in the sense of ignorance or disregard for life's richness inside. When we breathe shallowly in the chest, we're not at our best. We become prone to anxiety, stress, depression, fatigue, cardiovascular issues, and toxicity in our bodies. Move over blueberries. Our breath is our best antioxidant. If we are not breathing deeply, we are not ridding our body of toxins or experiencing full *joie de vivre*. SBA chapters would share breathing tools to enliven lethargy, elevate energy, and revive radiance!

Am I suggesting that breath is the next best thing to the internet? Actually, it's the other way around. The internet is phenomenal, but our breath provides access to our incomparable *inner*net. When we increase our capacity to take in oxygen and *prana* (the life force of the breath), we expand not just our lungs but our capacity to be present and increase our enjoyment of life. If we are feeling anxiety, depression, fatigue, shame, sorrow, fear, or paranoia, chances are we're barely breathing and definitely not experiencing "inspired life." Our inclination is to curl up in a fetal position, disappear under a mountain of blankets, or lie dormant in a cave, bed, or sofa. If you're hibernating for some rest and recuperation, that's one thing; if it's a consistent state of being, that's a formula for misfortune.

Luckily since breathing is our most basic mechanism for survival, our primitive brain makes sure we keep breathing, albeit in survival mode. The essential question is: *Do you want to merely survive, or do you want to thrive? Your response will determine how you breathe.*

The first two most important steps:

1. Set an intention to train your mind to watch your breath.
2. Focus your mindful awareness on *feeling* your breath.

Picture yourself for a moment lying low, because you're just not feeling the vim, vigor, and zest needed to get up and go. Shallow breathing has taken over, and you have no access to pep pills, caffeine, chocolate, or fire. *What to do?*

No matter your energy predicament, you always have an ever-ready "battery" in your breath. Simply bringing your awareness to noticing and feeling the physical movements of your inhales and exhales causes your breath to naturally deepen. Breath begets energy. Despite any challenge you may face, your own breath can act as a jumpstart to move from the cave to the mountain and "peak" experiences.

SHALLOW BREATHING	DEEP BREATHING
Upper chest	Lower belly
Often done through the mouth	In and out through the nose
Slumping posture	Erect open posture
Sedentary lifestyle	Active lifestyle
Low energy	High energy
Morose attitude	Joyful attitude
Unconscious breather	Conscious breather

Dr. George adds:

Our brain is constantly looking for danger and safety even when we are not aware of it. This means that all interactions, our environment, and even our internal dialogue (self-talk) is unconsciously being scrutinized in order to keep us safe. This scanning to protect us from danger is what neuroscientist Professor Stephen Porge calls neuroception, an unconscious process that takes place often activating our amygdala, which rests in our brain's limbic system deep inside the forebrain's temporal lobes. Although the smallest part of the brain, it plays a huge role in our lives, relationships, and reasons for shallow breathing. When I was a kid, I loved the TV series, *Lost in Space*. Whenever the ship's robot perceived danger, it flailed about and frantically screamed, "Danger, Will Robinson, danger." Our brain's amygdala acts as a radar, reminding me of that robot. When perceiving a threat, or feeling an emotional trigger, the amygdala emits a "red alert," thereby activating the sympathetic nervous system (SNS), propelling us into fight or flight mode and shallow breathing.

Without this ancient defense system, we might not be here. To survive, primitive people became "paranoid." Safety lay in assuming peril and venturing with extreme caution or not at all, rather than risk ending up as a tasty treat for a predator or a victim of a hostile clan. Imagine primates or early humans approaching a watering hole, food source, or potential mate with optimism and excitement, naïvely assuming a positive out-come. Their genes were less likely to make it into the gene pool.

Fear and hypervigilance kept our ancestors alive, which leads to the concept of negativity bias. We are wired to pay more attention to the negative, dramatically coloring how we view the world, ourselves, and our relationships. This is exem-plified in couples research findings; for every perceived neg-ative interaction that occurs, five positive ones are needed to balance or cancel it out. This 5–1 ratio illustrates the profound significance and attention our unconscious negativity bias places on hurtful, scary, and angry behaviors or interactions. Psychologist Rick Hanson, author of *Buddha's Brain*, states, "The brain is like Velcro for negative experiences and Teflon for positive ones."

Some of the most powerful interventions to calm the amyg-dala are breath awareness and practices, meditation, and pro-gressive muscle relaxation. At the heart of each of these tools is the breath. It can most quickly change our state from "Danger, Will Robinson!" to "All is calm—breathe easy."

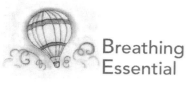

Breathing
Essential

Simply bringing awareness to feeling the physical movement of our breath naturally deepens our breath and helps calm our amygdala.

BLIPP

Watch your breath. Become aware of where and how you feel the physical movements of your breath in your body.

chapter six

Proactive vs Reactive

Gifts of Presence and Executive Functions

Whenever you take a conscious breath, you make a deposit for your health. And these deposits add up. Every moment of breath awareness is a deposit—a deposit as significant as gold. You probably have a savings account already for retirement or those "rainy days." Imagine creating a savings account for your health that doesn't cost a cent but just takes conscious, slow, deep breathing!

Let me put on my investment-broker hat for a moment. We usually breathe between 20,000 and 60,000 breaths a day. All or the great majority of these breaths are unconscious because most people don't think about their breath unless they can't breathe (not the most opportune time). With Western science proving the substantial benefits of conscious breathing, more people are paying attention. Each breath adds up, and before you know it you have a powerful investment and "reserves" for those times in life that compel "withdrawals."

You may wish to create a ledger and keep track of how much time you spend making "major" deposits. Examples could be playing a wind instrument, any exercise class, dancing, running (whether on a track or after your child), walking, biking, etc. Each activity benefits your respiration whether you are aware of your breathing or not. However, paying attention to your breath while you engage in the activity will greatly enhance the benefits.

You may ask, "Why would paying attention make it any better?"

Ahhhhhhhhhh! The answer: *presence*! Our bodies crave our presence. They call out, asking, begging, beseeching us for our attention. But sometimes the only way we "hear" our bodies is when they get sick, the illness "aching" for our awareness until finally we can't help but pay attention. Being proactively present to our bodies before becoming ill is a gift in the form of nourishment and nurturance that benefits us on all levels.

Dr. George adds:

How to be proactive? All of the conscious choices we make to support our well-being, whether physical, mental, or emotional, are referred to in neuroscience and psychology as executive functions—the ability to plan, organize, and implement our goals and tasks. Essentially this ability to manage our emotions, control our impulses, self-soothe, delay immediate gratification for better rewards in the future, and adapt to various interpersonal and intrapersonal realities is based on our ability to *self*-regulate.

Choosing to make Breath Literacy's Instant Power Practices (BLIPPs) an integral part of our lives, while remaining disciplined in their applications, are examples of applying executive functions. For example, we set our "intentions" to develop breath awareness and deeper presence in our bodies. Setting an intention, which is part of the job description of the prefrontal cortex (PFC), facilitates the mobilization of psychological, emotional, and energy resources, and directs them toward a specific goal. This conscious, directed mobilization activates various brain areas to work together and make our intention happen.

Think of it as a symphony where the conductor (the prefrontal cortex) is skillfully orchestrating a delicate balance of different instruments to create a melodious musical score. The conductor sets the intention to produce beautiful music (such as peaceful presence) and goes about working with the musicians (various areas of the brain and nervous system) to increase their ability to play and perform well together (proactively deepening presence in the present moment to help lessen reactivity in the future).

Our bodies are founts of wisdom, intuition, and intelligence. If we learn to more fully *inhabit* them, they can more easily alert us to any imbalances and let us know if something is needed right at the get-go.

James Joyce in *Ulysses* describes a character, Mr. Duffy, as living "a short distance from his body." Most people function this way. Our bodies are vacant while our minds are dwelling someplace in the past or future. In order to be proactive for our health and well-being, we need to "come home" to our bodies more often. And fortunately, in the vehicle of our breath, there's a "taxi" always waiting to bring us into "the now"—with no meter running to boot.

Our breath can serve as our GPS. Bringing awareness to it immediately takes us home from however faraway our thoughts projected us in time or place. There's no place like home!

I'll use the analogy of a house whose owner only visits once in a long while. With the owner gone and unaware, numerous troubles can begin to develop. Cute little dandelions proliferate and begin to break up the pavement. The small hole in the roof turns into a gaping cavity. The minor faucet drip becomes a plumbing disaster. The hairline crack in the foundation spreads until the wall begins to crumble. Critters congregate, creating colonies, webs, and nests.

You get the picture: A home needs to be inhabited, and our bodies require our attentive presence to help alert us to imbalances, ailments and "intruders" at the get-go. Hans Weller MD, asks, "Nearly every physical problem is accompanied by a disturbance of breathing. But which comes first?"

Conscious breathing is the most basic form of maintenance we can perform for our flesh-and-blood homes. Consistent, conscious breathing is not just maintenance but rather significant "home improvement." Consistent, conscious, optimal breathing (employing executive functions) over time can feel like upgrading from a home that was a shack to a carefree condo, or even a mansion.

What is consistent, conscious, optimal breathing?

Consistent conscious breathing is being persistently aware of the actual physical movement of our breath. This can be as straightforward as knowing when we're inhaling, and when we're exhaling. It's really quite astounding how simple that is, but simple doesn't make it easy. The key is practice.

Optimal breathing can be defined as the best / most correct way to breathe, which in any point of time promotes the highest forms of health, harmony, and well-being for the whole person—body, mind, and spirit.

Breathing optimally is both an art and a science. Part of the art is to find creatively consistent ways to bring our awareness inside, to noticing our breath. With continual practice, we feel more deeply the differences between our inhales and exhales. We know that just watching our respiration deepens and lengthens our breath. We get better with practice—concentration develops, and our ability to hold focus on the sensations of the breath increases. These neural pathways deepen and become neural "highways." With consistency, our proficiency and the benefits we feel soon expand exponentially.

Staying with the metaphor of inhabiting and caring for a "home," this comparison chart shows what consistent, constant "maintenance" fosters: [read left to right]

IN THE HOUSE . . .   *IN THE BODY . . .*

- Increased ventilation and air flow
  - *Expanded lung capacity*

- Strong and sturdy foundations, wall structures, and roofs
  - *Robust engagement of all cavities of the lungs and all respiratory muscles*

- Premier performance and longevity of all home appliances
  - *Heightened functioning of organs and glands*

- Heating and cooling systems that operate at their best
  - *Regulated emotions with the ability to be both energized and calm*

- Fresh groceries consistently taken in and garbage consistently taken out
  - *Fully oxygenated blood with fully released carbon dioxide*

- A house that is consistently cleaned, repaired, and refurbished
  - *Homeostasis with all body systems working at their best*

- TV / WIFI / satellite connections with the strongest signals
  - *Optimum mindful awareness and clarity of thought*

- Flourishing relationships in the home, neighborhood, and community
  - *Increased connections of body, mind, and spirit*

Conscious, optimal breathing is the most essential form of maintenance and renovation we can perform for our "homes." Health guru Dr. Andrew Weil asserts, "If I had to limit my advice on healthier living to just one tip, it would be simply: Learn how to breathe correctly." The rest of this book explicitly explains how to do this to proactively enhance your health and enrich your life.

In the "savings account" of well-being, we want you to amass a fortune.

DEEPENING TIPS: In any posture, let your hands and / or arms reflect the motions of your breathing. Perform each for a minute or more. Examples:

1. With palms up, rest hands in your lap. Now let the inhale raise the palms up about six inches and lower them on exhale.
2. Change to palms down on the exhale.
3. Inhale raising arms all the way up in front of you. Exhale, lowering them to your sides.

As you breathe, explore moving your arms in different ways to open your chest and naturally lengthen your breath.

Please visit www.BreathLogic.org for examples and routines.

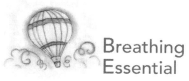 Breathing Essential

Awareness of your breath and breath practices must become daily routines / rituals.

BLIPP

Program yourself to be present in your body and breath as soon as you wake up, many times throughout the day, and when you prepare for sleep.

chapter seven

Calm those Nerves!

Understanding the SNS and PNS

Dr. George adds:

It's all about our nervous systems.

I'd like you to meet Bill. He loves to fish and decided to catch dinner. Feeling relaxed and breathing normally, he watched the sun sparkling on the waves. The furthest thought from Bill's mind was turning into a meal himself. However, seeing a shark rise out of the water takes his breath away. His heart races, blood pressure dramatically increases, liver releases glucose, eyes dilate, bronchioles in the lungs expand for more oxygen, digestion and reproduction processes halt, and his bladder empties. (Let's be practical; when fleeing from a giant fish, [or predator in the Serengeti], who needs extra weight to slow you down?)

What is happening? Bill's sympathetic nervous system (SNS) has kicked in, and he is in a state of fight or flight, the body's natural response to a perceived threat—or in Bill's case, a very real threat. In the limbic system of his brain, the ever-vigilant amygdala sends a dispatch to the hypothalamus, which messages the pituitary gland, which in turn alerts the adrenal glands that he needs to mobilize his resources for survival. This hypothalamic / pituitary / adrenal axis (HPA) results in the adrenal glands releasing adrenaline, noradrenaline, and cortisol. Because of this biochemical action that diverts mechanisms devoted to homeostasis into mechanisms for staying alive, Bill becomes ready to fight or flee.

Bill escaped becoming a feast because his body effectively mobilized his SNS fight or flight response to hightail it back to shore. Now he's lounging on the beach, quite content; respiration, heartbeat, blood pressure, digestion, and reproductive processes have all returned to normal, and he feels relaxed.

Are we not amazing creatures? This ancient "security" system has allowed humanity to survive. Designed to be adaptive and short-lived though, this age-old defense system has found new challenges in the twenty-first century "jungles." It is important to note that our body does not differentiate between a perceived threat or real threat. When the amygdala (neuroception) senses danger, whether it's a lion, tiger, or bear, or a problem with a boss, finances, or the kids, the SNS is activated and the fight or flight response kicks in. We can understand how this state, when long-term, compromises all the systems in the body, especially the immune system, wreaking havoc on our health and well-being.

Let's examine the sympathetic (SNS), and the parasympathetic (PNS) divisions. In the SNS fight or flight response, sympathetic nerves direct more blood to the brain and muscles that result in

- increased heart rate / blood pressure / sweating
- alertness / pupil dilation
- widened bronchial passages
- strengthened autoimmune system

The PNS rest and digest phase results in
- slowed heart rate / reduced blood pressure / nourishment
- increased digestive and endocrine gland activity
- relaxed sphincter and gastrointestinal tract
- sexual arousal / healing and regeneration of the body

The SNS inhibits the PNS. It is *catabolic*, meaning that significant bodily resources are utilized in the service of defense (perceived threats), and it wears down rather than builds up or nourishes our body. Again this is normal, healthy, and adaptive unless we cannot turn it off, as in trauma or chronic stress.

The PNS is *anabolic*, meaning that bodily resources are used to build and repair, which helps the body rest, digest, and regenerate. Remaining in a parasympathetic state much of the day, which breath awareness and BLIPPs cultivate, will allow the body to heal and nourish itself.

:

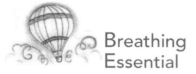

Breathing Essential

Our loved ones will appreciate when our breath takes us / keeps us in PNS (parasympathetic) dominance.

BLIPP

Become aware of what is currently causing you stress, and consciously become aware of your breath as you think of these things.

chapter eight

Your Greatest Treasure Lies Within

Home Sweet Home

Dr. George adds:

I provide workshops on stress, compassion fatigue, burnout, trauma, and posttraumatic incident procedures. In each of these trainings, I teach breath. Our breath is buried treasure that, when utilized, will replenish and heal. Since many participants come from diverse backgrounds (humanitarian, police, military, civilian, and numerous nationalities), I get some pretty quizzical looks when I talk about the importance of conscious breathing in our lives. I tout it as a main way to manage our nervous systems. Essentially I share what we teach in this book, that through conscious control of our breath, we can shift states (physiological, emotional, and psychological), thereby empowering ourselves with greater flexibility, resilience, and options.

Some people smile and clearly resonate to what I am sharing. Others look at me as if I'm speaking Greek or Swahili. Nevertheless, I persevere in the face of significant doubt until they can personally experience the prodigious benefits.

The Journal of Traumatic Stress published a study research-ing breath techniques utilized for American veterans with a post-traumatic stress disorder (PTSD) diagnosis from wars in Iraq and Afghanistan. The study utilized a powerful set of breathing techniques, which when practiced regularly, helped people with significant trauma symptoms feel safer in their bodies. The research indicated that controlled breath techniques reduced anxiety, startle responses, and helped with other reactions.

There is a huge amount of pain in the world. According to the Anxiety and Depression Association of America, approximately forty million American adults—almost 20 percent of the popula-tion, have an anxiety disorder. The National Institute of Mental Health (NIMH) estimates that in 2016, 16.2 million US adults had at least one major depressive episode. The US Department of Veterans Affairs (VA, 2018) released statistics that approximately twenty veterans commit suicide every day. The World Health Organization reports that over 300 million people worldwide suffer from depression and indicate that "Depression is the lead-ing cause of disability and is a major contributor to the overall global burden of disease" (WHO, 2018). With the repercussions of the worldwide COVID-19 pandemic declared in 2020, these numbers are exploding. There is a lot of suffering in the world.

Numerous studies show that specific breathing techniques support positive changes in psychological states. Here are just a few.

1. Stanford University School of Medicine researchers have found that nerve cells in the brainstem connect breathing to states of mind. (Affairs B.G., 2017).

2. A different study (Michael Christopher Melnychuk, 2018) discovered that how we breathe affects levels of noradrenaline in the brain, which at optimal levels can facilitate growth of new neural connections. According to the authors, "The way we

breathe . . . directly affects the chemistry of our brains in a way that can enhance our attention and improve our brain health."

3. In an excellent article by Zaccaro, et al., regarding conscious control of one's breath, the authors state, "Psychological/behavioral outputs related to the above-mentioned changes are increased comfort, relaxation, pleasantness, vigor, and alertness, and reduced symptoms of arousal, anxiety, depression, anger, and confusion." (Andrea Zaccaro, 2018)

Thich Nhat Hanh, peace activist, Zen master, author, poet, and advocate for breath awareness, is known as one of the greatest spiritual leaders of our time. His book, *At Home in the World*, illustrates the importance of breath in day-to-day, mindful living, illustrating the power of breath for managing our nervous systems.

During the First Indochina War, he was traveling as a young monk in a remote area of Vietnam to visit Bao Quoc Temple, located where many battles occurred between the French and Vietnamese Viet Minh resistance fighters. Gunfire, corpses, and fear were commonplace.

Near the temple, a French soldier hailed him, not to harass him, rather to inquire about an occurrence that had deeply impacted him. Hearing that Viet Minh were in the temple, the soldier's patrol went to find them. They approached in the evening, loudly shouting and stomping around. The soldier related that usually upon entering an area, people ran away in terror, but the temple appeared empty. This soldier turned on his flashlight and much to his surprise viewed 50–60 monks sitting still in silent meditation. The monks did not react in any way.

Thich Nhat Hanh explained, "They weren't ignoring you; they were practicing concentrating on their breath—that was all."

The soldier related how he was profoundly moved by this

experience. Their calm peaceful presence caused him to feel deep respect toward these monks, in effect shifting his perspectives about the Vietnamese and the war itself.

A second story touching me deeply relates to the topic of managing our personal nervous system. During the Vietnam war, Thich Nhat Hanh was sent by plane to evaluate consequences of a flood. At the airfield he encountered an American officer—a young man sent to a foreign country at war to risk his own precious life and potentially take the lives of others. Out of compassion, the monk asked, "You must be very afraid of the Viet Cong?"

As a result of that comment, the American soldier reached for his gun and demanded to know if he was Viet Cong!

Suddenly in an intense situation, Nhat Hanh realized his remark had invoked fear. Before coming to Vietnam, American military were warned that anyone, regardless of age or occupation, could possibly be Viet Cong. Grasping that this soldier could shoot him out of fear, the monk immediately slowed and deepened his breath, calming his own nervous system, and from this nonthreatening state, also calmed the nervous system of the soldier. Speaking with a gentle and soft voice, hoping to convey empathy for all victims of the war, Thich Nhat Hanh explained how a flood was the reason for his trip to Da Nang. The American soldier slowly took his hand off his gun.

The monk recounted later, "If I had acted from fear, he might have shot me out of his fear. By taking care and speaking in a mindful way, both of us were able to continue on our journey with a little more understanding between us."

Thich Nhat Hanh continues, "Mindfulness must be engaged. Once we see that something needs to be done, we must take action. Seeing and action go together, otherwise what is the point of seeing." Witnessing the devastation of the war prompted him to act to bring peace and end the war. As a result, he was exiled.

Thinking about the past, and home he could not see, was very painful. However his practice of mindfulness was a way to survive, live in the here and now, and feel the wonders of life in each day. He affirms: "The expression, '*I have arrived, I am home*' is the embodiment of my practice . . .

"I no longer suffer. The past is no longer a prison for me. The future is not a prison for me either . . . I am able to arrive home with every breath and with every step."

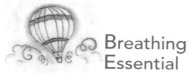

Breathing Essential

Our breath takes us within, helping us to "settle in" to our true home, a refuge that frees us from mourning the past and fearing the future.

BLIPP

Periodically, but especially if you feel disturbed or ungrounded, as you inhale, tell yourself, "I have arrived," and as you exhale, "I am home."

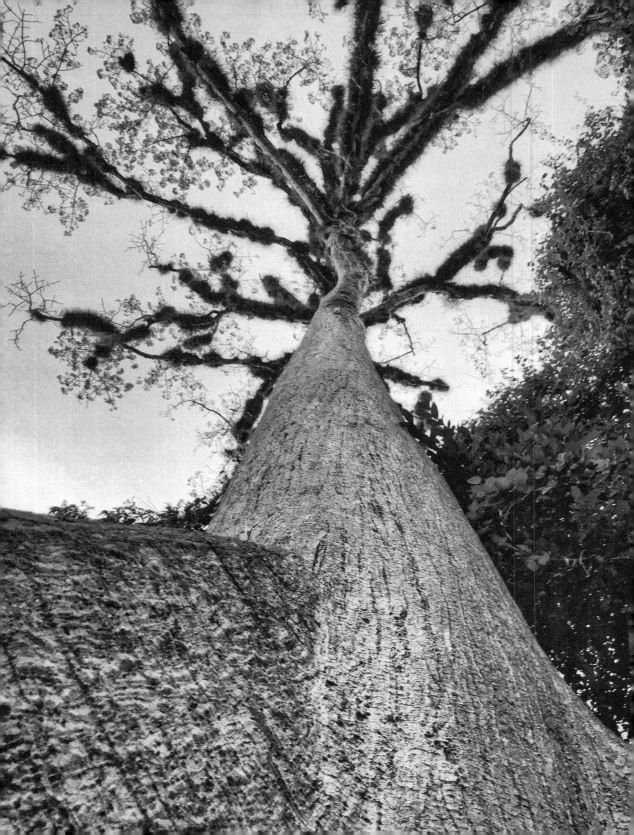

II

setting the groundwork

chapter nine

The Nose Knows

Foundational Breath Science

"A person should just as soon
breathe through their mouth
as eat through their nose."

• Yogi Ramacharaka in *The Science of Breath* •

Just as the nose is not meant to ingest and digest food, the mouth is not meant to filter and warm air. In yogic breath science, nose breathing is fundamental. As we take a breath (through the nose), the air becomes warmed and filtered by nose hairs and mucous membranes that trap miniscule particles of allergens, debris, germs, and other pollutants, making it fit to enter the delicate alveoli of the lungs.

The warming apparatus of our respiratory system is genius. The air in our lungs is 98.2 degrees, so the airways through the throat and nose are warmed as we exhale. Thus the inhale begins to be warmed upon entrance to the nose, immediately conditioning the air for its journey to the lungs. If we inhale through the mouth, we bypass this acclimatizing mechanism, which can be a great shock to the lungs in chilly climates. Yogi Ramacharaka adds that breathing through the mouth is a major contributor to colds, bronchitis, other respiratory ills, and a host of diseases. Our noses, whether like buttons, beaks, or honkers, huge or delicate, askew or straight, are not mere facial adornments.

Have you ever noticed that people in different areas of the globe have various "Mother Nature nose jobs"? Indigenous populations living in colder regions have longer noses in order to adapt better to warming the air in frigid temperatures. Inhabitants from warm desert environments also adapted longer noses because of the need to filter out desert sands. Those from balmy climates on all continents possess shorter noses.

No matter where you live or what size nose you have, it is imperative for optimal health to breathe primarily in and out through your nose. This habit begins at birth with the need of the infant to nose breathe while breast-feeding.

Here is a list of just a few essential reasons. Nose breathing . . .

- augments olfactory sense for enjoyment, emotional connection, survival,
- catalyzes antibacterial molecules to purify air/strengthens the immune system,
- helps prevent the inflammation of respiratory organs, colds, bronchitis, and pneumonia,
- keeps the nasal passages open (a disease preventative),
- interacts with olfactory nerves to stimulate the brain,
- regulates sleep patterns/reduces snoring,
- reduces the chance of sinus infections/helps balance the PH of the blood,
- lowers the heart rate (parasympathetic receptors in the nose),
- improves balance/increases brain wave coherence,
- enhances meditation,
- decreases anxiety/nourishes the central nervous system,

- alerts us to "fishy" or suspicious smells, and
- helps us "smell the roses."

DEEPENING TIP: Bring awareness to the sensations of the air entering and leaving the nose.

Osteopath Dr. Robert C. Fulford wrote in *Touch of Life*, "Remember: always try to breathe through your nostrils and not through your mouth, because air must contact the olfactory nerves to stimulate your brain and put it into its natural rhythm. If you don't breathe through your nose, in a sense you're only half alive."

Trekking in the high Himalayas and Andes presented me with lessons on nose breathing. I began to understand directly how utilizing my nostrils rather than my mouth enabled much deeper, consistent breaths. Ironically, I could cover more ground if I regulated my movement to my ability to keep breathing through my nose. Sometimes it felt like the classic "Tortoise and Hare" story: the hare being a mouth-breather and the tortoise—a nose-breather.

I noticed Sherpas breathing through their noses. For them, breath and presence were everything. Despite heavy loads on their backs and sometimes even barefoot, they maneuvered their cargoes so gracefully while moving steadily. Trekkers sometimes rushed past, mouths open and panting. The Sherpas just kept their pace, often passing by the resting sprinters.

After all these accolades for nose breathing, let's discuss when to engage mouth breathing. In daily life, breathing through the nose is vital, but specific situations can call for mouth breathing with powerful results. Remember that our brain affects our breath, but our breath also affects our brain. Inhaling through the mouth can engage parts of our brain's limbic system that are connected to stored emotions that we usually don't want to conjure up in our everyday life.

However, certain conditions can benefit from mouth-breathing therapies. Holotropic, rebirthing, and transformational breathwork play significant roles in catalyzing emotional healing by utilizing mouth breathing. In very specific circumstances, with knowledgeable facilitators, these forms of breathing enjoy great success in initiating powerful energy releases, discharging trauma, and promoting healing and well-being.

Sprinting may elicit mouth breathing on the exhale and also the inhale. Think of the breathing women do while giving birth. And the sublime breathing of long notes during singing and chanting. Music teachers point out that normal breathing typically involves shallow breaths using only the tops of the lungs. Singing involves the diaphragm and entire lungs in deep breathing. Another experience activating the diaphragm and often the mouth is the blissful breathing that can occur during orgasms.

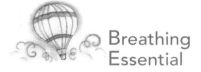

Breathing Essential

Breathing in and out on a regular basis through the nose is foundational to breathing optimally.

BLIPP

Close your eyes and focus on the feeling of the air flowing in and out at the tip of your nose. Engage this practice periodically throughout your waking hours.

chapter ten

How Are You Connected?

Posture and Grounding

When I was a young child, my mother used to remind us seven kids and my father of a memory from her days of nurses' training. She was studying at a small, Midwestern hospital where the head physician, Dr. William Delaney, proclaimed excellent posture—the "greatest preventative medicine" anyone could practice.

When the vigilant doctor walked the halls and encountered nurses standing or walking with even the slightest slouch, he came up behind them, and in a type of vertical karate chop, thwacked the side of his hand into the middle of their backs. This action instantly prompted the "angels in white" to press their chests forward while rolling their shoulders back and down, shoulder blades pressing in toward each other. Good posture was not good enough—it needed to be excellent.

Thankfully Mom never karate-chopped us, but she did carry out the role of "posture patrol," never permitting slumping or slouching. She and Dad both had excellent posture into their nineties, never stooping, and appearing much younger than they were. I've come to appreciate Dr. Delaney's postural idiosyncrasies as I've realized how ahead of his time he was in regard to preventive medicine and how essential postural bearing is for optimal breathing and overall health.

Dr. Delaney would be quite distressed to witness the epidemic of slouching and "hanging heads" these days, especially in children. In a "kinetic chain," the habit of a hanging head, for any reason, leads to rounded shoulders, curved spine, concave chest, tucked pelvis, and many other postural and physical problems.

If we slouch persistently, we cannot breathe fully, or properly distribute oxygen and release carbon dioxide. This means . . .

- our skeletal system is weakened, *which means* . . .
- our respiratory system is not functioning at its best, *which means* . . .
- our cardiovascular system is under strain, *which means* . . .
- our circulatory system is weakened, *which means* . . .
- our nervous system is challenged, *which means* . . .
- our digestive system is not operating optimally, *which means* . . .
- we're not metabolizing like we should, *which means* . . .
- we're not eliminating well, *which means* . . .
- our immune system is imperiled, *which means* . . .
- our vital organs are compromised, *which means* . . .
- we are aging prematurely, *which means* . . .
- our well-being is in a downward slumping slope.

Homeostasis and optimum well-being depend upon everything being connected. This downward spiral caused by poor posture can take us quickly, or slowly and insidiously, into a state of ill health.

Common complaints often derive from or are exacerbated by poor posture:

- aches and agonies of joints (hips, backs, knees, etc.)
- neck strains, kinks, and cricks

- tenacious tension headaches/painful pinched nerves
- nagging numbness/wretched range of motion
- sagging sore shoulders/consistent constipation
- absence of elegance, ease, and energy

A major reason yoga has achieved its evidence-based status as beneficial for health is because of a focus on the spine and correct postural alignment. There are styles of yoga for all ages, strengths, and flexibilities—even chair and bed yoga.

It takes some gumption to stand or sit up straight when everyone around us is comfortably slumping. It might feel satisfying to slump now if that is our habit, but those with straight spines will feel the benefits of better health as they age.

Compare yourself to a tall tree or a high building for a moment. The most important criterion for maintaining structural bearing are roots and a strong foundation. Like building any edifice, we construct our posture from the ground up. Grounding, establishing a firm foundation and connection with the Earth, is essential for posture and a secret for feeling more stable and energetic. Sometimes this is as easy as:

- becoming aware of how your feet are placed on the ground,
- walking barefoot on the earth when you can,
- imagining there are roots extending from the soles of your feet going down into the earth, or
- imagining/sensing your breath flowing down through your torso, pelvis, legs, and feet, connecting you firmly with the ground.

Grounding and postural elegance can become an innate ability like riding a bike. We begin to assimilate a type of body poetry and symmetry into our being. My dear friend, Susan, always carries herself in this way. She told me that as a very young child, her grandfather required her sisters and her to practice walking with glasses of water on their heads. Another elegant-postured friend balanced books. No matter what your age, it's not too late. I've watched many elders seem to grow inches just by looking forward instead of down, and teens transform their personas and exhibit confidence and self-esteem just by straightening up.

DEEPENING TIP: Keep your head and torso aligned over your hips. When walking, (especially up a hill) lead with your legs, engaging your core, not your upper torso.

There's icing on this cake. When we bring conscious attention and intention to posture and grounding, we experience more than physical benefits. We become more centered, balanced, and empowered immediately. In a popular TED Talk, Harvard researcher Amy Cuddy says, "Our bodies change our minds." She demonstrates the psychological differences between slumped postures and powerful, erect, grounded postures, and how they influence our lives.

If your work involves long periods of standing (clerks, construction workers, cooks, hairdressers, maintenance employees, medical personnel, teachers, wait staff, etc.), awareness of posture and grounding will likely help you to feel better, with more energy, at the end of your shift.

In her TED Talk, Isabelle Allende recounts Sophia Loren's reply to a reporter's question, "Why do you look so good?"

"Posture," she immediately responded. "My back is *always* straight." Then she added, "And I don't make old-people noises."

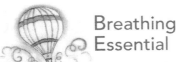

Breathing Essential

Grounding and excellent posture are the foundation for excellent breathing and excellent health.

BLIPP

Begin programming yourself to become aware of maintaining excellent centered posture whether standing, sitting, or moving.

chapter eleven

The ABC's of Breath Literacy

Awareness, Balance, Connection

To provide a complete course on Breath Literacy, we'll stay on the subject of foundation a little longer. To acquire literacy and develop fluency in any "language," we must start at the very beginning to integrate fully the building-block ABC's. From decades of studying, exploring, applying, and sharing wellness techniques from ancient and contemporary traditions and practices, I've observed three significant, common attributes.

In similar and diverse ways, the core of their essence and effectiveness are the ABC's: Awareness, Balance, and Connection.

AWARENESS	BALANCE	CONNECTION
attentiveness	equilibrium	union
mindfulness	stability	bonding
consciousness	solidity	rapport
responsiveness	equanimity	flow
wakefulness	poise	relationship
strength	strength	strength

DEEPENING TIP: Reflect for a moment on how these words (Awareness, Balance, Connection) apply to you personally, and how each can equate to strength in a distinct manner. Perhaps take a few minutes to write about them.

Can you recognize how each of the ABC's is unique, yet all function together in a powerful synergy? This short exercise emphasizes these dynamics. As you read this list, please bring your awareness to your posture and grounding (PG):

- Notice where your feet are. Are you solidly connected to the ground? (Even at the top of a skyscraper, there's a ground down there, and you can connect to it with your awareness, posture, and breath.)
- Do you feel the connection of your head to the sky? (Even in a basement, there's a sky up there, and you can connect to it with your awareness, posture, and breath.)
- Do you feel your weight balanced in your torso and feet, between front to back, and side to side?
- Can you become aware of the physical movement of your breath and differentiate between the feelings of inhale and exhale?

Savor this awareness. Savor the feeling of the flow of your breath. Relish sensing nuances of physical and energetic strength. If you like, relax and follow these sensations deeper into your body.

Ahhhhhhhhh! Could you feel that, as your awareness deepened, your sense of presence and calmness increased? Author and Zen teacher, Peter Matthiessen, revealed, "In this very breath that we now take lies the secret that all great teachers try to tell us."

According to *anapanasati*, a core breath meditation of Buddhism, "Breathing and mindfulness become one, two sides of the same coin. Awareness of breath reminds us to be mindful, and awareness of mindfulness reminds us to breathe."

Even if becoming aware of your breath is the only practice you ever do, as the core of mindfulness and meditation, your life will reap benefits. This is a sublime, time-honored practice that continually strengthens your consciousness and enhances your overall well-being. You can do it anytime, anywhere, while wearing anything from formal wear to your birthday suit.

If you don't feel anything right away, that's okay. For many people who may have experienced different types of trauma or pain, this doesn't come immediately. I assure you though, with practice and time (one breath at a time), it will. And it will change your life. I could share pages of research, facts, and stories to try to influence you, but the practice itself will convince you.

Western science used to postulate that, after a certain age, our brains could not be changed. With the studies of neuroplasticity, we know that our brains can continually create new neural pathways that physically change brain cells and foster change in our behaviors. Focusing awareness on our breath; knowing and *feeling* when we're inhaling, and knowing and *feeling* when we're exhaling is a foundational, yet master practice that teaches us how to experience "the power of now"—not living in the past or the future, but in the gift of the present. Moment by moment. Breath by breath.

DEEPENING TIP: Breath awareness turns any waiting time into practice time.

With repetition over time, some of the benefits practitioners notice:

- deeper calm and presence / greater ability to focus,
- increased lung capacity with greater oxygen flow,
- more balanced lengths of inhales and exhales,
- a tendency to breathe diaphragmatically,
- heightened attention to posture / feelings of stability and support, and
- deepened sense of intimacy with self, others, and the environment.

One way to cultivate Awareness, Balance, and Connection is to be conscious of "being present" where your feet are. Whether you are sitting or standing normally, in a golf stance, tennis-serve, one-leg balancing pose, skate blade skimming over ice, ballet slipper pirouetting, or tiptoeing through the tulips: *imagine breathing into your feet!*

Balance with your breath by keeping the inspirations (taking in) and expirations (letting go) steady, even, and flowing. This inner balance flows out into other areas of your life, helping to create outer balance between doing and being, work and leisure, time for yourself and time for others, etc.

Breathe into your eyes! We cultivate balance with sharp eye focus. Deepen connections of body, mind, and spirit by focusing your mind on your breath (spirit) flowing in your body. After you have connected inside, connect outside to how the earth and sky/heavens are supporting you. For a moment, perceive your connection to every living being.

DEEPENING TIP: Engage these practices/visualizations before any activity to let your "doing" emanate from the strengths of each ABC. Relish the empowerment.

One of my most significant teachers of the ABC's was a man I met in Guatemala. An acupuncturist, herbalist, tai chi and qigong master, James had studied many years in China. When he did tai chi, he did not *do* it—he embodied it! He was it. James believed that we needed to do a practice at least one hundred times before we could begin to make it our own. This is a way of turning the ABC's of the practice into muscle memory and a body/mind/spirit connection producing a moment of exquisite unity; for example, when a skater, dancer, or athlete performs a dazzling feat that lasts only one to several seconds but is done with a timeless presence and innate understanding of oneness.

Whether yoga, tai chi, qigong, ballet, hip hop, figure skating, hockey, tango, tennis, golf, weightlifting, walking, standing, or sitting, consciously incorporating the ABC's of Wellness will improve the performance of any activity.

Dr. George adds:

Like the breath, the vagus nerve is a vehicle of Awareness, Balance, and Connection between the body and mind via the neural regulation of our organs. This nerve is the largest nerve in the human body, starting in the medulla (base of the hind brain) and meandering through much of the body, ending in the gut. Essentially the vagus nerve is related to the parasympathetic nervous system, PNS / rest and digest, and functions as a "brake" on the sympathetic nervous system, SNS / fight or flight. This concept of a "brake" of the SNS is important to understand more fully.

When our neuroception (scanning for danger) determines that our internal environment (thoughts, feelings, needs) and external environment (job, relationships, outside world) are safe, the vagus nerve in effect applies the brake pedal of our nervous system and states, "We are safe to let our guard down and be present with ourselves and others." However, when our neuroception experiences our internal or external world as potentially unsafe, the "brake" comes off and the SNS kicks in.

Picture Bill (chapter 7) lying on his bed, miles away from his harrowing episode fleeing the shark. Although the incident happened months earlier, suddenly that memory pops into his mind and the razor-sharp teeth appear right in front of him. Since his brain doesn't differentiate between a real or perceived threat, he feels his body again physiologically preparing for flight or fight. Bill immediately becomes aware that his state has shifted from a sense of safety, pleasure, and calm, to fear, danger, and anxiety. This awareness is the first step in consciously controlling his physiological, emotional, and psychological states.

Bill has been practicing BLIPPs. BLIPPS cultivate awareness and engage the vagus nerve to "apply the brake" and stop his sympathetic nervous system's fight or flight mechanisms from taking over. The breath sends a message to the vagus nerve that says, "Hey, buddy, that was in the past, you are in the now and all is well." Instead of catapulting his body into the stress response for unnecessary reasons, Bill engages one of the many BLIPPs mentioned throughout this book and returns quickly to the PNS state of "rest and digest," feeling safe and calm.

We are safe–BRAKE ON	We are in danger–BRAKE OFF
• Internal and external environments are peaceful and calm.	• Internal and external environments are at risk (real or perceived).
• We can be present with ourselves and others in relationship.	• We are on edge and triggered.
• We stay parasympathetic.	• We go into fight or flight and relationship dynamics are difficult.
	• Sympathetic kicks in and dominates.

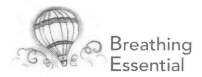

Breathing Essential

You can imagine and intend breathing into any part of your body to bring energy and kind attention to that area.

BLIPP

List whatever activities resonate with you, and look at how consciously cultivating and applying the ABC's (Awareness, Balance, and Connection) can enhance their practice.

chapter twelve

Breathing Mojo, Starring the Three S's

Soften! Smile! Sigh!

The bestseller, *All I Really Need to Know I Learned in Kindergarten* by Robert Fulghum, shows that effective wisdom doesn't need to be complicated or unusual, and often takes us back to the basics. In mindfulness training, we are asked to continually cultivate "beginner's mind." We are urged to explore information as if we are learning it for the first time. I invite you to try this as you read on to see how these S's can enhance and empower your life.

SOFTEN. Allow your eyes to close, softening your eyes. Soften all of the muscles around your eyes. Consciously let go of any tension you are holding in your belly. Soften your belly.

Ahhhhhhhhhhhhhh! Did you feel like you were melting?

Without realizing it, we tend to hold so much tension in our eyes—staring at computers, cellphones, TVs, and other close vistas. Taking a few moments to close our eyes, allowing them to relax, helps release tension throughout our body.

A dear friend, Bonnie, an emergency room nurse, experienced a death-defying car accident on the California coast. After work one day, her sporty maroon Datsun made twelve complete revolutions down a long, steep ravine. With the first roll, she willed her body to go limp "like a rag doll." While counting each surreal, slow rotation, she directed herself to consciously soften every part of her body. Her medical savvy side knew too well that in crashes and calamities, holding tension in the body serves to produce more trauma and broken bones.

Her rescue team couldn't believe anyone survived the flattened car. Back in an emergency room, a patient this time, she received stitches but had no broken bones, and was able to walk out the door. Bonnie relates, "Wearing my seat belt helped, but it was my ability to let go of the urge to tense up that made the difference, perhaps even saving my life."

Martial artists agree with Bonnie. When we tense, we tend to hold our breath. We become stiff and brittle. When we consciously remain soft, our breath and life force are still flowing, softening, cushioning, and protecting.

DEEPENING TIP: Inhale through the nose and exhale as slowly as you can through the mouth with a gentle *SSSS* sound, feeling the softening as you let out the air while gently contracting your abdominal muscles toward your spine. Allow your next inhale to be a relaxed expansion of your belly.

SMILE. Bring a soft smile to your face and feel that smile in your eyes. Soften your eyes. Consciously let go of any tension you are holding in your belly. Soften your belly. Smile to your belly.

I know this is an unusual request. Not something you'd hear in boot camp. However, if would-be warriors smiled to their bellies, it could end up lessening casualties or, at the very least, help manage stress. Some of the most fierce martial artists do this. (Taoist master, Mantak Chia, suggests smiling to all of our organs.)

Continue to breathe, soften, and smile to your entire body. When we bring a gentle smile to our face, we relax facial muscles. Our brain interprets this as being safe, calming our limbic system and causing dopamine, endorphins, and serotonin to release in our bloodstream. We end up feeling more relaxed, happier, and less stressed. Our bodies give us a rousing round of applause. Mother Teresa of Calcutta said, "Peace begins with a smile. Smile five times a day at someone you don't really want to smile at, at all. Do it for peace."

If possible, take a moment to close your eyes and really feel what's happening inside you. Author of *The Tao of Natural Breathing*, Dennis Lewis, recommends, "Breathe through your smile into your whole body. . . . Let the warm light of your smiling awareness and breath, touch, and awaken every cell of your body."

Now bring a full-on grin to your face. Yup, ear to ear. Bring it on! Studies show that the act of smiling triggers your left frontal cortex, the happiness center of the brain, releasing the "feel good" hormones that act as our body's natural pain relievers and produce positive physiological changes all throughout the body/mind. Photographers, dentists, and interviewers agree, smiles always make anyone more attractive. Smiles are a free facelift. Try something right now. Smile as you hold your breath. Now smile as your breath flows. Feel a difference?

DEEPENING TIP:
1. In your mind smile to someone you love. Feel them smile back at you.
2. In your mind smile to a stranger. Feel them smile back at you.
3. In your mind smile to someone with whom you feel conflict. Feel them smile back at you.
4. In your mind smile to the entire world. Feel the whole world smile back.

SIGH. Have you ever caught yourself or others sighing for what seemed like no reason? Or perhaps the reason was quite obvious from the sound and length of the sigh? Short sighs of mild irritation or long, loud sighs of exasperation? Languid sighs of boredom? Earnest sighs of yearning? Perhaps the different type of sigh conveying satisfaction, wonder, deep pleasure, or unbridled ecstasy?

Sighing is a natural reflex—inherent wisdom in our body that helps us release tension, frustration, and stress, and conversely deepens benefits of enjoyment. The longer exhalations generated by sighing cause reverberations of the vocal cords, thus turning on the brake of the vagus nerve, sending the signal to the heart to slow down. Deep sighs of letting go soothe the nervous system and help our bodies discharge detrimental emotions. Sighs of pleasure, like the ones we emit when eating something scrumptious, stroking a pet, making love, or receiving a massage, release powerful hormones like dopamine into our blood stream.

In *The Fine Art of Sighing*, novelist Bernard Cooper eloquently describes this powerful breath: "Poised at the crest of an exhalation, your body is about to be unburdened, second by second, cell by cell. A kettle hisses. A balloon deflates. Your shoulders fall like two ripe pears, muscles slack at last. . . . It's a reflex and a legacy, this soulful species of breathing."

Sighhhhhhhhhhhhhhhhhhhhhhhhhhhhh

Try this, or at least imagine, please. Put on your empathy cap to allow the feeling of replicating each sighing sound below. Don't be shy. Inhale through your nose and let the exhale release the specific experience:

- Short sigh of mild irritation / Loud sigh of full exasperation
- Languid sigh of boredom / Earnest sigh of yearning
- Contented sigh of satisfaction / Awe-inspiring sigh of wonder
- Pleased sigh of deep gratification / Voluptuous sigh of sensuality

DEEPENING TIP: Many people try to stifle their sighs. Knowing how beneficial they are, make it a practice to let yourself sigh often and fully. When your sigh is deep and full, it fosters a deeper and fuller inhale, allowing you to optimally utilize the "magic" in the air.

Dr. George adds:

Softening, smiling, and sighing are three excellent BLIPPs for helping to manage stress. The term STRESS is interwoven into the fabric of Western society, warning of its dangers to our health. We see references to stress in newspapers, magazines, and academic courses. Most of us struggle with stress a great deal and realize the negative impact it can have on our lives. Stress is sneaky. It can creep up on us without warning, and soon we find ourselves exhausted, emotional, ill, and prone to making mistakes.

By breaking down the different types of stress, we can more clearly see how Breath Literacy is a powerful component of any stress-prevention program or treatment regimen.

Hans Selye, often called the father of stress research, was the first person to begin developing a comprehensive theory regarding stress. In the 1940s, he was the first to posit that many illnesses have a stress-related component. Basically, stress is the result of something that throws our psychological, emotional, and/or physical systems out of balance. According to research by the Physicians Council on Stress, 60–80 percent of all illness may have a stress-related component. Some specialists believe this is an underestimate.

Stress can be negative but also has a positive side. Selye coined the phrase, "Stress is the spice of life." Stress can have exciting, motivating, and life-enhancing effects on us—called *eustress*. Preparing for an important event, sports, marriage, dating, interviews, and performances are all stressors that can add to the quality of our lives. In reality, eustress helps us learn, adapt, and change.

However, when most of us talk about stress, we refer to negative stress and its adverse effects. In the case of a car accident, robbery, experiencing a violent incident, a betrayal, illness, financial struggles, disappointment in how our lives have turned out, work problems, divorce, etc., stress is distress.

As already noted, our stress response was designed to be short-lived. When an animal or early human in the jungle or the Serengeti was attacked and survived, they shook themselves off and went on with their lives. Their physiology returned to parasympathetic; they were no longer in fight or flight mode. Modern life has many more dangers, e.g., school shootings, injustice, war, crime, viruses, social distancing, and so much more. Our bodies are designed for short-term stressors, not ongoing long-term stress. Consider the types of stress:

Acute stress is short term. We encounter this all the time, a traffic jam, a minor car accident, or a spat with a loved one that is resolved quickly. The body returns promptly to a parasympathetic state without accumulating the significant reactions or symptoms that often manifest with chronic, long-term stress.

Episodic acute stress manifests when acute stress is experienced frequently. Type-A personalities can be vulnerable to episodic acute stress as they tend to be competitive, handle a lot of responsibility, and are often in a hurry. Those with this type of stress often take on more responsibility than they can handle comfortably.

Traumatic stress, which may or may not result in post-traumatic stress disorder (PTSD), is the result of exposure to incidents outside the range of normal human experience, e.g., robbery, rape, imprisonment, systemic forms of marginalization and dehumanization such as racism, sexism, sexual and gender discrimination, domestic violence, and war. This can be experienced personally or by witnessing it happen to someone else. Hearing about something horrible happening to a loved one also fits in this category.

Chronic stress is built up over time and results in the regular release of stress hormones (adrenaline, noradrenalin, cortisol) that eventually wear out the body, adversely affecting the immune system, cardiac functioning, cholesterol, blood pressure, etc. Our bodies were not meant to be on constant Red Alert. Chronic stress is quite dangerous because our bodies are essentially in a sympathetic state far too often.

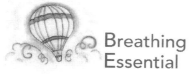

Breathing Essential

Softening, smiling, and sighing develop mojo, ease the flow of breath, reduce stress, and promote optimal wellness.

BLIPP

Program yourself so that you intermittently soften, smile, and sigh all throughout your day, but especially when you begin to feel stressed.

chapter thirteen

Whole Lotta Shakin' Goin' On!

Maximum Benefits for Minimum Effort

"A person's age is not measured by number of years
but by flexibility of the spine."
• Yogic wisdom •

Late one night while watering the little garden of our desert home
in the Middle East, I discovered that workmen had left a "treasure"
in our alley: an extension ladder so lightweight I could maneuver it!
Knowing they'd be back to pick it up, I thought I'd borrow it overnight to paint a wall in our living room.

My husband George thought I was crazy, but knew that when I
get something into my head there's usually no stopping me. "Are you
sure you want to do this now at 10:00 p.m.?"

"Absolutely! We only have the ladder until morning, and I'm not
tired." Resigned to my determination, he went up to bed.

I put on music and climbed up the ladder to stretch painter's tape
along the eighteen-foot-high ceiling. Halfway done, the not-well-latched

ladder began to flatten out. In a split second that seemed to last forever, I was pitched toward the hard stone floor, jutting out my left hand to try and break the fall. The surreal experience began.

Awakened by the crash, George was almost in as much shock as I as we gazed at my hand, strangely dislocated from my arm.

We arrived three hours later at the medical center amidst a sea of exotic robes and covered faces. Two men held me down as two doctors tried to realign my hand to its wrist without anesthesia. I was not shy in belting out screams of excruciating pain tempered by "fire breathing" that sounded like I was birthing a very large mammal. The worried expressions on the doctors' faces intrigued my husband. (My screams didn't faze them, but my breathing did.)

"Don't worry," he assured them. "She does this."

Afterward, my arm strapped on a board, I lay in a waiting room and began to focus on my breath and body. First I noticed a slow shiver. Then my lips started to quiver, my jaw to quaver, my hands trembled, my legs shuddered, shoulders rocked, and soon every part of me was shaking uncontrollably. Because I have a daily shaking practice, I sensed how important this was and, instead of trying to stifle the movements, I gave myself over to them completely.

Shake, rattle, and roll! For several minutes, my entire body vibrated to some deep inner wisdom that took me for a ride, as my nervous system seemed to go berserk. George was about to call for help when the shaking began to lessen, and then halt, conveying me out of shock to a destination of balance. An exquisite deep stillness and peace replaced the movement, the trauma completely subsided.

I found others had similar episodes. A dear friend, Janet, described how after a major surgery, her body went into spontaneous shaking which she intuitively felt was part of the healing process. Lasting about fifteen minutes, she questioned at one point, "Will this ever end?" Nevertheless surrendering to it completely, she was eventually transported to a place of peace and calm. Though certainly unorthodox behavior, such shaking is quite normal for some people and animals. Shaking is a practice in qigong and in kundalini yoga, and is quite prevalent in nature. A gazelle in the Serengeti becoming a near-miss meal for a leopard will shake itself off and then be able to go about its day. Dr. Henry Emmons, author of *The Chemistry of Calm,* shows video of this scenario in many of his presentations.

Any self-respecting dog or cat would never get up after being sedentary without boosting life force by stretching and/or shaking. From gentle bouncing up and down, mild loosening, wild gyrations, and everything in between, there are shaking practices to fit your mood and music. The aim is to help you deepen your breathing, alleviate stiffness, boost your immune system, and augment overall well-being. If you have time for only one physical practice a day, let it be "shaking."

My predilection for this practice is based on time-tested and time-honored benefits (over thousands of years actually) and maybe a little laziness. For me shaking is not something I have to do, it's something I want to do because (add gongs to the bells and whistles): *This BLIPP has maximum amount of benefits with minimum amount of effort.* Before we know it, our breath is deepening, flowing to our extremities, and every cell is being bathed in life force. Our attention becomes more present in our bodies as we glow with vibrant energy. Say goodbye to rigor, and hello to ease, as our breath is freed from the constraints of the torso. Stiffness succumbs to flexibility, our spines become suppler, and our bodies and minds can respond with greater resilience to the winds and stresses of life.

You see, stress leads to tension. Tension leads to stiffness. Stiffness leads to:
- sore joints/aches and pains/poor circulation/lethargy,
- sluggish functioning of organs and glands/lowered immune capacity, and
- proclivity to break bones (usually wrists, ankles, and hips as we get older).

Rigidity in our body can lead to rigidity in our thoughts, attitudes, and behaviors. Martial artist Bruce Lee advised, "If nothing within you stays rigid, outward things will disclose themselves."

DEEPENING TIP: Are you a teacher, presenter, trainer? Studies show that sedentary spectators do not absorb information like active audiences. Go ahead! Shake 'em up! They'll love you for it.

CAUTION: As with any new exercise program, you may wish to check with your doctor that this is right for you.

SHAKING PRACTICE
1. Come first into a very modified *"HORSE STANCE."*
- Place feet shoulder-width apart, with toes and heels equal distance from each other, your weight distributed evenly over both feet. Take time to settle into inhabiting your body.
- Allow your knees to softly bend, sinking your sacrum downward.
- Relax your shoulders back and downward as you press the crown of your head upward, lengthening the back of your neck.
- Feel yourself grounded, supported by the Earth beneath your feet and connected to the heavens through the crown of your head.

2. Start with GENTLE BOUNCING.
- Begin to very gently start bouncing up and down while loosening.
- You may "pick up the reins" and imagine riding your steed. After a short time let go of the reins and relax hands and arms by your side.
- Close your eyes, focusing on your breath, allowing the gentle movements to continually aid letting go of tension throughout your body.

3. Increase to *VIGOROUS SHAKING*.

- Begin to loosen fingers, hands, wrists, elbows, shoulders, gaining momentum until you are vigorously shaking your entire body. Explore movements with your hips, raising your arms overhead, bending the torso, shaking your head, jowls, etc. *Enjoy*.
- In the final minute to thirty seconds, give it all you've got. Smile.
- *PERFORM* for one to ten minutes.
- TO END: With eyes closed, come gently into stillness, take one to ten additional minutes to focus inside, noticing the effects of the practice.

DEEPENING TIPS: Close your eyes to focus more fully on feeling your breath and the flow of energy in your body. *Put on your chosen music, and make it fun!*

Benefits:
- Enhances the flow of life force / energizes / relaxes and warms.
- Aids functions of all the body systems, organs, and glands.
- Promotes detoxification / boosts immune system.
- Strengthens spine and bone marrow / improves lymph flow.
- Burns calories / loosens joints / reduces cellulite / tones sagging tissues.
- Encourages grounding / fosters deeper breath and body presence.
- Increases longevity / clears the mind / rouses you out of a rigid rut.

Telling you that shaking is an empirical, time-honored practice is not enough. Several years ago, I attended, with one hundred other people from around the world, a groundbreaking Breath Immersion Conference at Omega in New York.

The first thing that presenter Dr. Richard P. Brown (clinical professor of Psychiatry at Columbia University) had us do was shake. This was important to me for several reasons: First I revere shaking—I've been doing it and teaching it for several decades. My energetic, flexible friend, Jan, in her eighties, considers morning shaking her longevity practice. My dear colleague, Karyn, shakes to relieve depression. BreathLogic board member and CEO coach, Debby, and her husband Jeff, shake several times a day to energize and increase flexibility. I have felt in my bones how beneficial it is, yet I had never seen or heard any academician share it or talk about it. Dr. Brown feels that shaking is one of the most important techniques he can share. He has used it with all kinds of populations including refugees suffering from untold traumas. I loved this!

For a time, I resented the reluctance of the scientific/academic world to accept at face value the benefits of many ancient practices: yoga, qigong, mindfulness, meditation, breathwork, shaking, etc. Easterners embraced these techniques for centuries, but many Westerners require studies and proof before even trying them. My husband George and I used to get into tiffs about this.

For some reason though, hearing Dr. Brown talk about how "shaking" helps soothe the nervous system *did* make it more substantial for me, and *I got it* why it's so important to have studies and substantiation. If this is what some people need in order to try something—please bring on the research!

George needed the verified studies on the benefits of mindfulness in order to become a daily practitioner. Even though Breath Literacy practices are new to the West, I was able to help convince him with a few but growing number of authenticating studies (and bribery, if I'm honest) to try them.

Ahhhhhhhhhhhhh! As blues artist Jessie Mae Hemphill sang, "Shake it, baby!" Soothe your nervous system, and think beautiful positive thoughts.

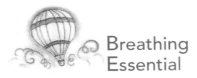

Breathing
Essential

Gentle bouncing and shaking deepen the breath and provide maximum benefits with minimum efforts.

BLIPP

Make gentle bouncing / shaking a get-out-of-bed routine. Bounce / shake in the afternoon when you've been sitting too long or need an energetic pick-me-up.

chapter fourteen

DO YOU MIND?

The Power of "Now" and The Power of "Belly"

Now that we've consciously shaken things up, let's look at consciously settling in with The Power of "Now":

Dr. George adds:

In 1979, Jon Kabat-Zinn, PhD, professor emeritus of medicine at the University of Massachusetts, founded the Center for Mindfulness in Medicine, Health Care and Society, and the Stress Reduction Clinic. Mindfulness for stress reduction is now a known and respected methodology. Kabat-Zinn defines mindfulness as a conscientious discipline revolving around a particular way of paying attention to the present-moment awareness of life with an attitude of nonjudgment.

Mindfulness is a practice that requires cultivation. This is a way of being in the world, fully aware of moment-to-moment experiences, interactions, feelings, and sensations in a caring, loving, and nonjudgmental way. Kabat-Zinn states, "If you are breathing, then there is more right with you than wrong."

Mindful breathing is at the heart of being present in the world and in our relationships with others and ourselves. In *Full Catastrophe Living*, he states, "Our bodies are joined with the planet in a continual rhythmic exchange as matter and energy flow back and forth between our bodies and what we call the environment. One way this exchange of matter and energy happens is through breathing. With each breath, we exchange carbon dioxide molecules from inside our bodies for oxygen molecules from the surrounding air. Waste disposal with each out breath, renewal with each in breath."

Dr. Ed Hallowell offers reasons why mindfulness begins with the breath:

- "The breath doesn't try to get anywhere." We breathe in and out. We don't try to do it perfectly. We just are being.
- "The breath teaches us steadfastness." By using our breath as an anchor in life, we can calm our scattered minds and come back to our breath again and again, which cultivates resilience to be present in the moment.
- "The breath happens in the body." When we breathe calmly and gently, we are more likely to breathe into our bellies.
- "The breath isn't really that boring." A breath is like a fingerprint. Each is different. The sensations, duration, location, and texture of our breath are a surprise and adventure each time.
- "You don't breathe. The breath breathes." Observing our breath changes the relationship we have with ourselves. Letting our body breathe in its own way, simply allowing, observing, and appreciating is good training in all parts of life that we have little control over. The breath breathes us.

- "The breath invites us to rest and recuperate." Breath leads us back to the parasympathetic nervous system, rest and digest.

Mindful breathing takes us out of automatic pilot and brings us back to our "senses," offering more options for how to perceive situations, respond to challenges, and remain parasympathetic. As a way of being in the world, we can be intentionally present to our experiences in an open, nonjudgmental way.

The final part of mindful breathing is attitude. In *Full Catastrophe Living*, Kabat-Zinn initially listed seven attitudes to cultivate. Later he added another.

1. Nonjudging (Be an objective observer of one's own experience)
2. Patience (Cultivate tolerance and serenity)
3. Beginners Mind (See each moment as if it were new, a childlike view)
4. Trust (Self, body, emotions)
5. Non-striving (BEing and allowing rather than doing)
6. Acceptance (Surrender to what is happening in this present moment)
7. Letting Go (With each exhale, we let go)
8. Gratitude and Generosity (Big-heartedness)

Other authors have added compassion and kindness. All are interconnected and bidirectional. As we are kinder and less judgmental to ourselves, we may also judge others less. As we work to be more patient with ourselves, we become more patient with others. Trusting ourselves more, we are more likely to trust others, and so on.

Each of the attitudes represents an intention, a way of viewing the world, an image, and a feeling. For example, with gratitude: I commit to invite gratitude into my consciousness and hold it even if I am not feeling grateful. As I remind myself of things in my life that I am grateful for (my wife, health, passion for learning, even limited tennis skills) I experience feelings and images of my gratitude. As I hold this in consciousness, I am aware of my breath, for which, bluntly, I am eternally grateful.

We can use our breath as an anchor to exit acting from autopilot (reactive habit rather than conscious choice) and deliberately transport ourselves back to moment-to-moment awareness, bringing with it a nonjudgmental, caring, and compassionate attitude. In this way, mindful breathing is a bridge to mindful living.

Remember neuroplasticity—the brain's ability to rewire itself to change its structure and function? Essentially, what we feed (give focus to) grows, and what we stop feeding disconnects, unwires or, metaphorically speaking, dies.

We can change our thoughts, feelings, and responses and create new neural pathways or we can continue driving on our old highways and, through repetition, further reinforce our anxiety, anger, depression, or unhappiness. What we focus on strengthens. If gratitude, positivity, and kindness to self and others is what we focus on, that is what we strengthen. We fake it till we make it. Attention, repetition, and a patient, loving, and caring attitude toward self is the foundation for this change. We can recreate ourselves consciously. Our minds and breath change our brains, and our brains change our breath and minds.

The Power of Your Belly

One of the most important ways to accomplish these changes is through mindful attention to our bellies. If you've ever watched a baby's respiration, you've witnessed the remarkable little belly rhythmically rise fully on the inhale and lower on the exhale. This is our inborn way to breathe—engaging the diaphragm, our body's largest muscle. This beautiful, natural way of breathing is unlearned by most people as early as young childhood. Babies held by caregivers who are stressed, holding their breath or breathing anxiously in their upper chests, can pick this up by osmosis. Most people I work with have to relearn how to breathe diaphragmatically. I did.

It is of utmost importance that we relearn how to do it.

Unfortunately in our current society—actually for centuries, the belly has been given a bad rap. Whether men or women, we've sucked in our bellies. Men have been "belted in" and women have suffered from instruments of torture like corsets made with whale bones, cutting us off from our *haras*, a Japanese word meaning seat of life force and source of empowerment. You may have heard of this area referred to as *dantien* or core. Imagine for a moment that you are strapped into a corset—hold your stomach in as much as possible. Women who suck in their breath and bellies to narrow their waists have endured headaches, fainting, menstrual problems, miscarriages, poor constitutions and other ailments. For folly of frivolous fashion, we have cut off the power of our life force!

Holding in your stomach and still trying to breathe? How crazy is this?

Ahhhhhhhhhhhhhh, let your belly relax and notice how it naturally expands to take in the life force the inhale gifts you. *If we hold tension in our bellies, it's impossible for our mind or body to be relaxed.* Our sympathetic nervous system will be dominant while we consistently experience a mild-to-severe state of anxiety.

I've had many different breath teachers; some focused on Eastern practices—pranayama (prana=life force, ayama=to master, thus the science of how to master our life force), Taoist, qigong, or tai chi styles of breathing. Others focused on the physical aspects of breathing—Western respiratory science. Various teachers emphasized energetic, emotional, or spiritual facets of the breath.

One of my most significant instructors, Elizabeth, had the most amazing voice I've ever heard. I first listened to her "instrument" with my eyes closed. She started warming up with breathing. Her solo voice sounded like an entire room of yogis in India practicing *ujayyi* (the ocean-sounding breath). When Elizabeth started singing/toning, her range soared from the deep bass of chanting Tibetan monks to the high, pure notes of a choir of celestial angels. Her "concert" brought me to tears, and I knew I needed to study with her. Elizabeth stipulated that she only took students who first committed to a year of practicing deep belly breathing for at least one hour a day. I responded, "Absolutely!"

I took two weeks off work for intensive one-on-one sessions and then began the year of daily one-hour-minimum, Diaphragmatic/Belly Breathing. Usually in the morning, I put on an hour of soft music. I lay on my back with my hands on my lower belly, sometimes knees bent, other times not. I focused on feeling the physical movement of my breath as low in the belly as possible. When I first started, I could feel my breath in the thoracic and clavicular chambers of my lungs. After much practice, I was able to isolate my breath to only my lower belly and lower back. That's when *I really began to notice changes.*

Physically, I became able to sense my diaphragm, and then actually experience it move. After several months, I became aware of the processes of digestion and elimination. After about six months, I could tell when I was ovulating and also when menstrual blood was going to be released—experiences I had been completely unconscious of before. I had no idea they could even be perceived.

Mentally, I could be bored, my mind wandering, thinking about anything from the weather, to food, to sex. At times, forgotten images from the past, sometimes with accompanying emotions, appeared in my mind's eye. Finally, when my mind settled into its work of connecting my body with my breath (spirit), time took on different dimensions. Being focused in the "now" of each breath made time fly.

Emotionally, a variety of feelings, ranging from frustration, anger, sadness, and grief, to delight, peace, elation and empowerment, flooded over me. I sobbed, laughed hilariously, or felt numb, nothing, or nirvana. I allowed the emotions to flow; my directive was not to fixate on them. As much as possible, I remained focused on executing and feeling the isolated physical movement of each breath.

Intuitively, I connected more profoundly with a source of inner wisdom and knowing, cultivating greater ability to let go and trust.

Spiritually, I felt the breath as life force animating my body. Most of the time it was orchestrated by my volition; keeping my breath only in my lower belly (explicit instructions). Sometimes at the end of the hour, I continued lying there, effortlessly being breathed, feeling the serenity and well-being of connection to something so much greater than myself. The ability to trust blossoming into a divine nonchalance, realizing as philosopher, Alan Watts asserted, "We both breathe and are breathed."

For well over a year, I never missed a day, and I attribute significant self-transformation to this work. I literally found my voice, along with courage to make changes in residence, relationships, and work. Empowerment began to flow through my life in more trusting, cognizant, and creative ways. I realize that the mindful, fuller breathing catalyzed more mindful, satisfied living.

In the next two chapters we will more comprehensively explore the power of the belly and Belly/Diaphragmatic Breathing.

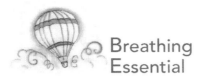

Breathing Essential

We strengthen what we focus on.

BLIPP

Practice breathing with and focusing on an attitude of your choice:

non-judging

patience

beginner's mind

trust

non-striving

acceptance

letting go

gratitude

generosity

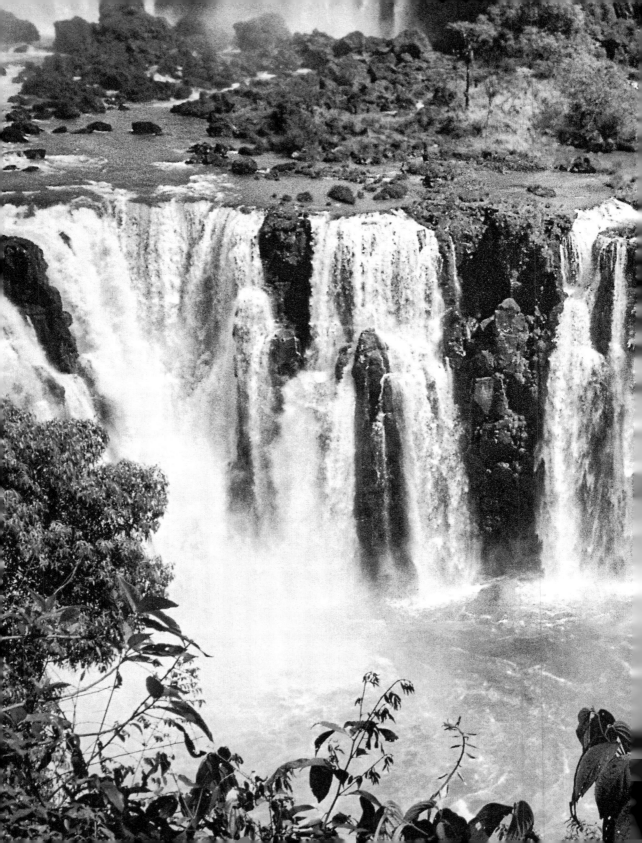

III

foundational breathing practices

chapter fifteen

Belly Up and At 'Em

Powering Up with Diaphragmatic / Belly Breathing

The science of yoga looks at the body as being inextricably connected to the mind, emotions, and spirit. They interface each other. We are physical, and we are energetic. The physical work of Diaphragmatic/ Belly Breathing brings positive ramifications for our emotions, mind, and spirit, as well as our body, resulting in a form of cleansing or purification.

On a physical level, we digest our food. Energetically we also digest—assimilating and eliminating—or not, what we experience mentally and emotionally in life. As our bodies store physical toxins, we also store mental and emotional toxins from our life's experiences.

One of my instructors described it as: "Breath is life. With any experience in life, ideally, we assimilate the aspects of experiences that serve us and help us grow into our energetic-being while eliminating those aspects that don't serve us." Psychologists and counselors refer to this as reframing, self-soothing, forgiving, letting go, etc. The alternative is that experiences "eat away" at us—mentally and emotionally at first, perhaps disrupting our sleep, perhaps later manifesting as an imbalance, pain, or disease.

My teacher explained: "Shit happens. If we're alive, it's bound to happen. How we deal with it is what matters. By living life, we're going to accumulate 'baggage' and produce 'garbage,' physical and energetic. Do we carry these burdens and debris with us all our lives unconsciously, or intentionally deal with them through therapy, exercise, prayer, dance, etc., and/or our breath?"

Conscious breathing is one of the most effective methods to make *shift* happen. We can become our own composters, counselors, therapists, and "house" cleaners. Cognitive therapy can be remarkable but it's essential to know we can also help ourselves. With deliberate awareness of the letting go and taking in of our breath, we can energetically digest, eliminate, and cleanse without having to know exactly what, when, where, why or how the "compost" happened. We just "take out the garbage" and let it go.

Our bellies are sources of wisdom (gut intuition), power, and stamina. It's as if we're battery operated. By breathing diaphragmatically, the diaphragm pushes down and the belly presses outward revving up our "battery." We connect to an inner source of energy that is physical, mental, emotional, and spiritual. During the months spent trekking in the mountains of Nepal and Peru, I came to understand this so well. Often although exhausted, I still had to climb a few thousand feet or more before encountering food and shelter. I garnered energy in four main ways:

1. Sitting with my back against a tree, breathing slowly and deeply in my belly as I imagined connecting with the life force flowing through the tree.
2. I ate an energy bar.
3. I performed the rapid, deep belly breaths of *Kapalabhati* (Breath of Fire).
4. I had a good laugh.

Have you ever wondered why laughter feels so exhilarating and energizing? You know the kind where you just can't stop and your belly aches afterward. Holding your belly in would be impossible. While laughing, we breathe diaphragmatically, exercising our inner organs and triggering the release of endorphins. Our breath becomes deeper and our brain receives more oxygen. "Feel-good" hormones flood through our cells and our body/mind glows. *Reader's Digest* knew it long ago with their regular section, "Laughter: The Best Medicine." It's the same with a good cry. As singer Joni Mitchell and others have noted, *"Laughing and crying . . . it's the same release."*

A good cry can be a release in more ways than one. When we allow ourselves to sob, our breath activates our diaphragm. Whether bawling or guffawing, we experience the physical benefits of deeper breathing, increasing the capacity of our lungs, engaging the lower back lobes of our lungs (where 60–80 percent of our blood supply waits to be oxygenated).

Here is another story about the power of Belly Breathing.

A lovely woman, Joan, had severe anxiety manifesting in agoraphobia. With big, soulful eyes filled with tears, she related her story. For ten years, she found it difficult and sometimes impossible to leave her house. The hardest thing for her was missing precious moments of her darling daughter's young life. In the mornings, Joan would tell her: "Honey, I'm going to be there today!" for the afterschool soccer match, play, or other event. As a devoted mother, she meant it. But in the afternoons, as she approached the door, her breath rushed into her upper chest, her heart pounded, and a full-scale panic attack prevented her from opening the door and leaving.

"If I'd only learned to breathe into my belly then, I wouldn't have lost ten years of my life!" Joan lamented to me. "Most importantly, years of my daughter's life! Just learning to belly breathe changed my life, allowing me to turn the knob and walk out the door."

If you've ever been in a state of panic, you understand what Joan went through. Panic induces the fight, flight, or freeze responses in the body, restricting the breath flow into the upper chest where the breath is held or becomes rapid and shallow. In these circumstances only a very conscious act of engaging the diaphragm can counteract the course of our body's well-oiled stress response.

DEEPENING TIP: Imagine a balloon inside your belly. As you exhale the balloon deflates. As you inhale the balloon inflates.

Physiologically, it is impossible to be in a state of full-on panic if we are breathing into our bellies. The physical act of bringing our breath low and slow, engages the diaphragm, stimulates the vagus nerve, and directs the brain to arouse the nervous system so that the PNS (rest and digest) dominates over the SNS (fight or flight) eliciting a relaxation response in the body. A panic attack cannot take over, and anxiety is kept at bay when this occurs. Simply and powerfully, belly breathing is a constantly accessible, life-changing tool.

Dr. George adds:
I first became aware of the distinguished career of Professor Steven Porge while training in trauma studies (2016–17). His book, *The Polyvagal Theory: Neurophysiological Foundations of Emotions, Attachment, Communication, and Self-regulation*, genuinely shifted how I view the role of the autonomic nervous system (ANS).

Historically, neuroscience conceptualized the parasympathetic and sympathetic branches as antagonistic, serving different functions and working at odds. However, the polyvagal model views these branches as working together in a fluid back-and-forth rhythm that supports health and well-being (strong immune system, good digestion, healthy heart, and sound sleep). Traditionally, the fight / flight, and freeze responses were both viewed as manifesting from the same neural circuit of the sympathetic nervous system (SNS). Professor Porge shows how the freeze response comes under the parasympathetic nervous system (PNS).

The polyvagal theory posits that the nervous system has three neural circuits that evolved at different stages of human evolution:
1. The social engagement system.
2. The sympathetic nervous system.
3. The earliest and most primitive, dorsal vagal complex, which is related to the freeze (feigning death, or immobilization) response.

As Laurie puts it:
1. We breathe easily in our bellies.
2. We breathe rapidly in our upper chests.
3. We hold our breath.

To illustrate the three neural circuits, Porge uses the concept of a street light:
• **Green**=safe (Our actions, thoughts, and emotions reflect safety, social engagement, and connectedness.)
• **Yellow**=possible danger (We are in fight or flight, with feelings of anger, fear, and a desire to act or do something.)
• **Red**=life-threatening (We are feeling helpless or hopeless and our dorsal vagal complex / reptilian brain immobilizes us.)

In a red state that our brain interprets as life-jeopardizing, we freeze, potentially disassociate our thinking and feeling, and often do not fully remember what occurs. Some people (like Joan in the above story) find themselves living in the red zone, in a state of immobilization which could mean dissociation—a state of "not being there." For example, many victims of rape describe that they left their bodies and hovered above the incident.

Two breathing techniques recommended by Professor Porge:
1. Diaphragmatic Breathing (Belly Breath)
2. A longer exhale than inhale (Relaxation Breath)

Breathing into the belly and long exhalations activate the parasympathetic vagus nerve, telling our body we are safe, there is no need to "act" right now; rather, be calm, relaxed, and present in the moment with oneself and others.

POLYVAGAL CHART

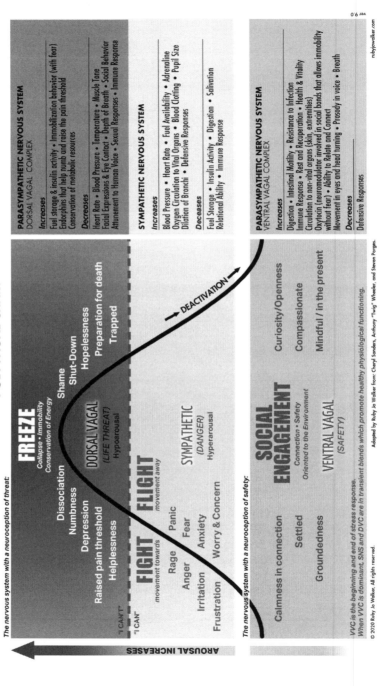

The nervous system with a neuroception of threat:

"I CAN'T"

FREEZE
Collapse • Immobility
Conservation of Energy

Dissociation
Numbness
Depression
Raised pain threshold
Helplessness

DORSAL VAGAL
(LIFE THREAT)
Hypoarousal

Shame
Shut-Down
Hopelessness
Preparation for death
Trapped

"I CAN"

FIGHT
movement towards

Rage
Anger
Irritation
Frustration

FLIGHT
movement away

Panic
Fear
Anxiety
Worry & Concern

SYMPATHETIC
(DANGER)
Hyperarousal

DEACTIVATION →

The nervous system with a neuroception of safety:

SOCIAL ENGAGEMENT
Connection • Safety
Oriented to the Environment

Calmness in connection
Settled
Groundedness

VENTRAL VAGAL
(SAFETY)

Curiosity/Openness
Compassionate
Mindful / in the present

AROUSAL INCREASES

PARASYMPATHETIC NERVOUS SYSTEM
DORSAL VAGAL COMPLEX

Increases

Fuel storage & insulin activity • Immobilization behavior (with fear)
Endorphins that help numb and raise the pain threshold
Conservation of metabolic resources

Decreases

Heart Rate • Blood Pressure • Temperature • Muscle Tone
Facial Expressions & Eye Contact • Depth of Breath • Social Behavior
Attunement to Human Voice • Sexual Responses • Immune Response

SYMPATHETIC NERVOUS SYSTEM

Increases

Blood Pressure • Heart Rate • Fuel Availability • Adrenaline
Oxygen Circulation to Vital Organs • Blood Clotting • Pupil Size
Dilation of Bronchi • Defensive Responses

Decreases

Fuel Storage • Insulin Activity • Digestion • Salivation
Relational Ability • Immune Response

PARASYMPATHETIC NERVOUS SYSTEM
VENTRAL VAGAL COMPLEX

Increases

Digestion • Intestinal Motility • Resistance to Infection
Immune Response • Rest and Recuperation • Health & Vitality
Circulation to non-vital organs (skin, extremities)
Oxytocin (neuromodulator involved in social bonds that allows immobility
without fear) • Ability to Relate and Connect
Movement in eyes and head turning • Prosody in voice • Breath

Decreases

Defensive Responses

© 2020 Ruby Jo Walker. All rights reserved.

VVC is the beginning and end of stress response.
When VVC is dominant, SNS and DVC are in transient blends which promote healthy physiological functioning.

Adapted by Ruby Jo Walker from: Cheryl Sanders, Anthony "Twig" Wheeler, and Steven Porges.

rubyjowalker.com

ver 9.0

TWO SCENARIOS

SCENARIO ONE:

Jessica was late again—willing the traffic to speed up had no result except to make her tense and her breath shallow.

A scowl on her face, she sat in the motionless car, her mind racing a hundred miles an hour, ruminating about everything she had to do: *pick up the kids, visit the nursing home, call the dentist, deadlines at work, clean up the latest mess, shop for dinner.*

As her breath came out in shallow, rapid gasps, an urge to scream and beat the dashboard rose up.

   "Aggghhhh! It's impossible to breathe!"

   Helplessness and Stress!

   "My life is an uncontrollable mess," Jessica bemoaned, "I might as well book my hospital room now!"

SCENARIO TWO:

Jessica was late again—accepting the traffic jam caused her to take a deep belly breath and let out a long sigh.

A gentle smile on her face, she sat in the motionless car, her mind slowing her breath, focused on staying present in the moment by watching her breath and soothing her racing mind's obsessive "to do" list by repeating the mantra "peace."

As her deepening breath moved lower into her belly, the anxiety and tension continued to dissolve.

   "Ahhhhhhh! The chance to just breathe."

   Empowerment and Peace!

   "No matter what the circumstances, Jessica rejoiced, "I have it in my power to stay calm, enhancing my well-being."

Is it really possible for experiences similar to Scenario One to metamorphose so easily into Scenario Two? Can we so quickly turn an out-of-hand, stressful situation into one of calm and control? The answer is unequivocally: *YES!*

The key is knowing how to change our breath before flight or fight takes over.

Practice Diaphragmatic / Belly Breathing

Lie comfortably on your back with eyes closed and both hands on your belly.

1. Focus inward on feeling the physical movement of your breath. Begin first by exhaling while contracting the belly toward the spine (as if you are squeezing your navel to your back).
2. The resulting inhalation is a natural extension outward of the belly. With this relaxed expansion, the diaphragm presses downward, aiding in the movements.

Benefits:
• Regulates physical and emotional states.
• Provides an antidote for anxiety and promotes tranquility.
• Increases energy and stamina.
• Massages inner organs and aids digestion.
• Strengthens grounding and body presence.

Diaphragmatic / Belly Breathing is so important to well-being that it is essential to practice it to the point where it becomes our **natural / default way of breathing.**

Expanding your belly does not mean you will get a big belly. Actually this breathwork will strengthen your diaphragm, your abs, and your core. For some people, this is a total shift in paradigm for how they breathe, even how they dress, and who they consider themselves to be. Breathing in the belly is foundational breathing and will create foundational changes.

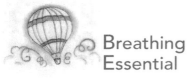

Breathing Essential

It is physiologically impossible to be in a state of full-on panic if we are breathing deeply in the belly.

BLIPP

If possible, perform belly breathing while lying on your back as a way to start your day before you get out of bed and when you prepare for sleep. Whether lying down, sitting, or standing, practice belly breathing often throughout the day. The simplest advice: Keep it **low and slow.**

chapter sixteen

Stressin' Out!

Make Stress Your Ally

"Fear less,
Hope more;
Eat less,
Chew more;
Whine less,
Breathe more;
Talk less,
Say more;
Hate less,
Love more;
And all good things are yours."
• Swedish Proverb •

In working with our breath, it's essential to thoroughly address the topic of stress. Stress normally reaps a really bad rap, and rightly so, yet stress is not all negative. Dr. George talked about *eustress*: short-term, beneficial stress that aids us in dealing courageously and effectively with the "winds" of life. In this chapter though, we deal with long-term, harmful, chronic stress that can lead to debilitation, disease, and demise. There's bad news but also good news. We'll start with the bad news and end on a very positive note.

Stress is in the news: big time! Countless studies relate that chronic stress is prevalent in our culture among not just adults but children too. Innumerable articles, blogs, podcasts, books, treatises, and tomes have been written about the insidiously serious, health-harming, and life-threatening effects of chronically stressin' out. Author and meditator, Natalie Goldberg wrote, "Stress is basically a disconnection from the earth, a forgetting of the breath."

When we are "stressin' out," we might feel like our poise, power, privacy, and precious possessions have been hijacked. But it turns out, it's just our amygdala. According to author, psychologist, and mindfulness teacher, Therese Jacobs-Stewart, "The neural cluster known as the amygdala cannot distinguish between real physical danger and an emotional threat. . . ."

Dr. George adds:

The body does not know the difference between a shark attack or a problem with the boss, children, mortgage, or traffic. If you perceive a situation as dangerous, fight or flight will kick in. Some people might call problems or worries about work, marriage, money, relationships, etc., paper tigers. This concept of a "paper tiger" was brought into English by Sir John F. Davis in his book, *The Chinese*, and was used to describe something (or someone) that appears to be dangerous, powerful, threatening, and scary, but in reality, is not.

Paper tigers can have profoundly adverse effects on our physical, mental, and emotional health when we give these thoughts or mental creations so much power, meaning, and reality, such that a failed deadline, bad test results, embarrassing situation, or fight with our partner feels to us like life or death.

I am defining a "real" threat as violence or imminent demise. Real threats are what the sympathetic nervous system was designed to address: life-or-death short-term threats. They are either over and we move on, or we are history. Our sympathetic nervous system was simply not designed to be activated most of the day. There are two ways to trigger danger in the brain, top down or bottom up. Paper tigers are top down (made up in our minds), and most imminent danger is bottom up (physical reality).

We may be caught in traffic, fearing that if we're late one more time, our job is on the line. This "paper tiger" and escalating anxiety (*Oh no! How are we going to pay the bills, put food on the table, send the kids to school, etc.*) makes our breath shallow in our upper chest, signifying danger to our amygdala. For many people affected by COVID-19, these anxieties felt like "flesh-and-blood tigers." Before we realize it, our brain is preparing our body to engage in battle or flee for our very lives. Stress hormones such as adrenaline and cortisol flood our bloodstream and brain. Adrenalin increases our heart rate and elevates our blood pressure. Our system stops digesting food and repairing cells. Blood is shunted away from our vital organs and propelled into our arm and leg muscles so we can attack, defend, or run. The negative bias of our reptilian brain acts as if "this is it"—survival is on the line, so there is no need to . . .

- digest the rest of our meal (Here comes indigestion, constipation, diarrhea, or stomach aches),
- repair cells (Say goodbye to graceful aging),
- fight germs, bacteria, or viruses when death is in the wings (Say hello to a weakened immune system),
- make a baby (Say farewell to fertility),
- have the kidneys filter the blood (There goes a healthy circulatory system),
- etc., etc., etc.

What makes stress insidious in our bodies is that long-term harmful effects may not show up right away. Later, autoimmune disease, cancer, or any number of illnesses rear their ugly heads. It is nothing to laugh about. But actually, this would be one of the best things that we can do: Laugh about nothing!

"Laugh about nothing?"

Yes, take the curative abilities of laughter seriously. When we don't feel like laughing at all is when we most need to laugh. It gets our breathing into our belly, which stimulates parasympathetic activity. Of course, it's more fun to react to something truly comical rather than to nothing, but our brains do not differentiate between responsive laughter or forced laughter. The physical act of laughing and the resulting Diaphragmatic / Belly Breathing releases feel-good hormones into our bloodstream, counteracting stress. Dopamine, endorphins, GABA, melatonin, norepinephrine, oxytocin, and serotonin, among others, serve to elevate our moods, access feelings of pleasure, reduce pain, diminish depression, create calm, aid focus, improve sleep, and help us age gracefully.

For centuries in India, people have gathered together for a practice of spending time crying, laughing, and in silence. Inspired by this, in 1995 Dr. Madan Kataria began gathering people in parks in India to participate in "laughter yoga." Laughter clubs all over the world began congregating people to chuckle, chortle, howl, hoot, and guffaw together. Each of these ways of laughing moves the breath into the belly and revs up our oxygen levels. Once we start laughing, it's easier to keep going. As Dr. Seuss wrote, "From there to here, and here to there, funny things are everywhere."

Now it's time for more positive news. We have abilities to become stress resilient with something as simple and as powerful as a laughing practice ten minutes a day. Read jokes, watch funny YouTube videos and comedies, or fake it until you make it. Here's icing on the cake: Ten minutes of deep belly laughter is work on your abs equal to 300 sit-ups. Really, what would you rather do?

DEEPENING TIP: Have you ever wondered why belly laughter feels so good? It's all in the breath, hormones, and activation of our relaxation response. Have you ever reacted to sad, stressful situations by breaking out into "inappropriate" laughter? "Ho Ho," says the innate wisdom of the body searching for release and balance.

I remember as a very young child with my little brother Tommy, listening over and over to a scratched recording of raucous laughter to which we continually hooted hysterically. Our mother would be going about her work but sometimes just had to stop and laugh along. Laughter is contagious and an excellent antidote to secondhand stress. Just as secondhand smoke can harm nonsmokers, being with others who are chronically stressed can upset our own well-being. Being with others who take laughter seriously can enhance our well-being.

While George and I were living in Cambodia, an exceptional yoga teacher, Isabelle, began working with very young women who had been sold to brothels at tender ages. Their experiences were impossible to fathom. When I met them, soon after they had been rescued, they reminded me of deer in headlights, homeless refugees, and prisoners on death row. They appeared shocked, battered, humiliated, and hopeless, their bodies housing unimaginable distress. As trauma expert Dr. Bessel van der Kolk wrote: *The Body Keeps the Score*. These girls were incapable of meeting another's eyes, let alone closing them to be consciously present inside, aware of their breath.

Isabelle worked with them for two years with vigorous ashtanga yoga with an assistant, Vannac, translating for her. She met their resistance, anger, shame, and revulsion with empathy, compassion, and the clear instructions to work their muscles in systematic ways that helped to release the trauma in their body/minds. These intensive, physical techniques began to help them feel again, cry, laugh, and slowly reclaim their bodies as their own and as a safe place.

Witnessing their transformation was phenomenal. After two years,

I was able to engage them fully in laughter yoga and deep mindfulness meditation. Their once-lifeless eyes were filled with joy and vibrancy as they burst into giggles, and then later stayed comfortably closed in the finding of sanctuary inside.

Vannac, Isabelle's translator and student, once a gang member, went on to become Cambodia's first national yoga teacher.

It's easy to laugh when we feel good, but it's when the world appears dim, that we can most benefit from laughter. Children normally laugh hundreds of times each day, and adults, only a few times. All we have to do to welcome laughter back into our lives is to make the decision and set the intention. Then laugh, whether "it" is funny or not. Our brains will release mood-elevating hormones either way.

Our point of power is that with our physical body (the way we breathe in our body), we can calm our mental and emotional states. Thich Nhat Hanh tells us, "Peace is your every breath."

- *Our bodies change our minds.* Breathing deeply strengthens neural pathways to soothe the amygdala and calm our minds. (*We feel peaceful.*)
- *Our minds change our behaviors.* When calm, we are not triggered to lash out, cortisol is not released. (*We act in a peaceful way.*)
- *Our behaviors change our outcomes.* If we don't lash out, there is no fight. (*Others react to our peacefulness with their own peacefulness.*)

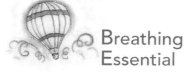

Breathing Essential

The easiest and most powerful way to perform deep Diaphragmatic / Belly Breathing is by laughing.

BLIPP

With hands on your belly, giggle or laugh for a full one to ten minutes. Enjoy this practice at least once a day.

chapter seventeen

Let Go and Be Happy

Raise Your HQ (Happiness Quotient)
to Lower Your IQ (Irritation Quotient)

"There is no duty we so underrate as the duty of being happy.
By being happy we sow anonymous benefits unto the world."
• Robert Louis Stevenson •

Who knew that by being happy we can help the world! (I had started to feel some guilt about being happy when I knew so many people were stressed and suffering.) When I first read the above quote, I was thrilled. It resonated with me, and became the impetus to study happiness, and increase my "HQ—Happiness Quotient" or ability to feel content and gratified with whatever life presented me. I read studies suggesting that often it's not the big stressors in life that mostly mar our contentment; rather it's those minor annoyances and irritants.

I learned that in order to sustain a high HQ, we need to maintain a low IQ—Irritation Quotient, or propensity to become easily aggravated. Just as tiny, buzzing, biting mosquitoes can spoil a glorious summer evening, small aggravations can begin to add up. Before we know it, they are "under our skin," morphing into chronic stress and eroding our happiness, harmony, and health.

An irritation can start as an inconsequential annoyance: someone fiddling with their hair, cracking gum, drumming their fingers on the table—any type of behavior that's prone to annoy, bug, or madden— someone asking too many questions, being cut off in traffic, not moving fast enough when a red light turns green. It can be another person's voice, gesture, action, or inaction.

If you're in a state of high HQ, you can easily overlook niggling sounds. But with a rising IQ, these noises can morph in your mind into clamors, worsen into commotion, and escalate into a full-scale horrific hullabaloo. You may feel like nails are scraping across a chalkboard next to each ear—and it's all "their" fault! What's there to do but respond with outrage?

I've been there. Not just outrage—justified outrage! I had a right to be irritated and stressed! And by God no one was going to take that satisfaction from me! Even though I knew all the negative physiological effects the stress was causing, the satisfaction of knowing I had a darn good reason for feeling it, made feeling it downright good and rewarding. But letting oneself go into an utter tirade always has negative repercussions. Therese Jacobs-Stewart writes in *Paths Are Made by Walking*: "This stew of stress hormones secreted when a person is upset takes hours to become reabsorbed in the body and fade away. In fact, it takes at least four to six hours and sometimes several days."

Such an episode occurred years ago, when I was traveling alone in India on a budget. I felt so accosted by men and barraged by tuk-tuk drivers; sellers of Tiger Balm, candy, hashish (and anything else you can imagine), beggars, children, and masses of humanity, it took every ounce of will power to stay halfway centered. Finally an incident with a hostel owner was the last straw. When he tried to withhold my passport, I stood up on a table and started to scream. It felt so good that I began to jump up and down (still on the table) while screaming louder and louder. Anyone watching surely thought I'd lost my mind.

I had definitely lost my mindfulness. I'd been stuffing irritations for too long. The "eruption" felt like freeing myself from a straight-jacket. I did get my passport back, but it was not one of my proudest moments. A few years later I was on the other side of a tantrum.

While working as a gate agent at the Minneapolis airport, I was in charge of a flight at the end of Concourse G. I implored my supervisor to hold the plane for a connecting passenger, a Mr. Jorgenson, arriving late, "miles away" at Concourse A.

She ruled, "No. The flight must go out on time." I waited until the last possible second but with my passenger nowhere in sight, I did as told and returned to the podium for post-departure work. Only minutes passed before I heard in the distance, panting breath and enormous-sounding pounding feet. An image of an attacking Viking (not the football player, the ancient warrior) came into my mind. Taking a deep breath, I braced myself.

Mr. Jorgenson rushed to the counter, barely gasping, "Did I make it?"

"I'm sorry, sir, the flight went out on time."

With a face red as a tomato, the poor, peeved passenger let out a wail (sounding like a war cry invoking Thor) followed by a barrage of four-letter words. Before my astounded eyes, this six-foot-plus man dressed in a suit threw his briefcase on the ground, followed by the length of his entire, long body. With arms and legs thrashing, he pounded the floor for a full minute, an anguished *"AARRRhhhhhgggg"* accompanying the pummels.

I did not think this was going to end well. My secondhand stress response had kicked in—flight, fight, or freeze? Should I run and hide in the jetway, call security, or remain immobilized behind the podium? My breath and brain chose "freeze."

Holding my breath, I watched transfixed, and then flummoxed as his fury abated. Transforming into a "gentle giant," Mr. Jorgenson got up and brushed himself off as if nothing had happened. Looking sheepish, or perhaps self-satisfied, he sighed and then very calmly allowed me to book him on a later flight.

Coincidentally, soon after this episode, I attended a workshop touching on research-based benefits of tantrums. The best tantrum engages both the body and the voice, resulting in deeper breathing and deeper letting go. That was definitely my experience in India, and also Mr. Jorgenson's at the airport.

Now think for a moment of how children are quite connected to the "wisdom of the body." When feeling deep frustration, they will naturally tantrum. With age, they're taught more mature methods of letting go of big frustrations. Methods perhaps more socially accept-able yet less effective in relieving the results of stress hormones creat-ing chaos in their little bodies, raising their IQs, lowering their HQs, and training them to stuff emotions.

In the science of yoga, and in Eastern medicine, emphasis is put, not only on the physical body, but also the "subtle body," what many people term the "energy body." We feel the effects of stress first in the subtle body. Imagine for a moment that these stresses or irritants are tangible: every time you feel irritated, a teeny, tiny "globulet" of guck forms. A massage therapist might experience them as knots. If they add up, they can begin impeding the flow of energy and important functions of major systems in the body, sooner or later, causing problems—big or small.

We can't always eliminate irritants, but we have the potential to eliminate our customary reactions. Common advice might be: "Take a breath and count to ten." This can be effective for some people. For others, this type of breath is high in the upper chest, strengthening the fight or flight response, and when the count reaches 3-2-1 they're ready to explode.

However, if we respond right away to a minor irritant and engage a "Letting Go" BLIPP—belly breathe, sigh, smile, laugh—it can dissipate before escalating from mere nuisance to unrestrained eruption. BLIPPs (especially daily shaking practice) help prevent irritants from building up and morphing into reactive anger that makes us scream, swear, throw things, slam doors, argue, fight, or pull out hair, stopping short hopefully before we torture, maim, murder, or go bald. Arun Gandhi, Mahatma Gandhi's grandson, teaches that the majority of violence in the world is not premeditated, but reactionary. As a child living with his grandfather in India, he learned that anger management—lessening susceptibility to become irritated—was essential to the path of nonviolence, well-being, and peace.

DEEPENING TIP: One way to slow down and halt the trajectory toward unintentional reactivity is to periodically practice a version of what the Mindfulness-Based Stress Reduction (MBSR) program calls "STOP."

S Stay present. (Sense where your feet are, grounding.)

T Take a breath. (Notice a full cycle of inhaling and exhaling.)

O Observe. (Experience your body, mind, and emotions.)

P Peacefully proceed. (Continue with greater calm and awareness.)

If in the O=Observe part, you notice you are feeling negative thoughts or emotions, take an extra moment and breathe with them. Acknowledge them. Even honor and thank them for letting you know you're raising your IQ. Maybe you need to make a pact with them that you will return and examine them later. In the meantime, *let go* with a long sigh, take a belly breath and more consciously proceed with what you were doing, feeling a little more peace of mind and being.

> Dr. George adds:
> We have been talking a great deal about psycho-physiological states and developing the skills and knowledge to change our state. I make it a habit to "STOP" and check in" with my body as frequently as possible. This "check-in" asks two things:

"Where might I be feeling tension in my body?" and "Where is my breath right now?" We often slip into sympathetic without realizing it.

An example, recently, Laurie and I were in a taxi and truly not in a rush. However the traffic was dense, and my body was reacting like "let's get this show on the road!" I was clearly in sympathetic and felt my body tense, my breathing change, and my impatient attitude become dominant. I stopped and did a brief body scan revealing I was tight in my shoulders, neck, and core. I began to visually let go of the tension by softening my muscles while slowing and deepening my breathing. Quickly my state shifted and I felt calmer and more appreciative of where I was in the moment, who I was with, and that all was well.

The point: we can learn to check in with ourselves regularly. This is a self-taught strategy, making letting go and shifting states much easier when the situation requires.

For many people, having to wait is one of the biggest irritations to erode personal peace and happiness. Examples:

- *Waiting* in traffic jams, for red lights, "Sunday drivers," construction . . .
- *Waiting* for an answer, result, diagnosis . . .
- *Waiting* for noise to abate (lawn mowers, horns, drills, music . . .)
- *Waiting* for computer updates, uploads, downloads . . .
- *Waiting* to talk to a real person when put on hold . . .
- *Waiting* in lines at a store, airport security, bank . . .
- *Waiting* for a meeting or appointment to start—or end . . .
- *Waiting* to be waited on . . .
- *Waiting* for life to return to normal . . .

Watchfully, wistfully, wearily, winsomely, wordlessly, warily, woefully, waiting! Aspects of waiting figure into the top life stressors: death, divorce, diagnoses, finances, careers, health, personal relationships, chronic illness, pregnancy, infertility, danger, and fear.

It can seem like we're always waiting for something or someone, and that there's nothing we can do about it. But thankfully we have the *BLIPP* power tools to "let go" and transform the feelings of irritation and powerlessness to those of peace and empowerment.

THE KEYS:

1. Employment of BLIPPs for positive reactions at the first signs of irritation.
2. Consistent proactive, preventative, health-enhancing practices.

In his book, *The Art of Happiness*, the Dalai Lama convinced co-author and psychiatrist, Howard Cutler, that happiness is not a luxury but the purpose of our existence; its achievement is scientific and requires discipline. Achieving happiness does not depend on events. Dr. George reminds us of our ability to rewire our brains. With mental practice we can create the ability to be happy most of the time. Bobby McFerrin simply sings, *"Don't worry, be happy."*

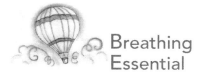

Breathing Essential

Every breath offers a conscious choice.

BLIPP

Use any waiting time for consciously applying posture and grounding (PG), Awareness, Balance, and Connection (ABC's), softening, smiling, sighing (3 S's), and low, slow belly breathing.

chapter eighteen

Nostrils: They Know

They Really, Really Know

"I'm getting a cold, I can't breathe at all, and we have no Nyquil!" George complained as he came in the door. "The training starts tomorrow. This could not have happened at a worse time!"

We were in postwar Kosovo, and he was facilitating a UN training that had been planned for months. There were no open-all-night drugstores where he could purchase cold medicine.

Here's my chance! I thought gleefully. George had heard my claims of not succumbing to colds. He'd actually seen me do it but never had the opportunity to experience it himself.

"Well, Hon, if you want, I'll help you," I offered, knowing that if ever he'd take me up on it, this would be the time.

"What do I have to do?" he inquired, looking quite skeptical.

"First you must clear your nasal passages for Alternate Nostril Breathing" I replied, probably way too cheerily.

"That would be a miracle," he countered.

"You'll see, it will work. However, you're going to have to put effort into it. Healing is based on bringing the body back to a state of balance. You're out of balance right now, but working with the currents of breath can bring you back to balance. Since this only hit you full blast today, you can counteract it. As long as you can clear your nasal passages and keep them clear, the cold can't take hold. Whoever said a cold has to run its course did not know about breathwork."

I thought back to a frigid, January day in Minneapolis where I was house-sitting in a very drafty artist's loft. The wind chill had plummeted the temperature to 60 below zero and I felt the beginning of a raging cold. The next day I was scheduled to give an intensive workshop on breath. *Oh yeah,* I thought, *I can't even breathe myself! Okay, time to practice what I teach.*

After brewing fresh ginger root tea, I attempted to unblock my stuffed-up nose by doing several hours of different types of Alternate Nostril Breathing (some of this I did very consciously and some I did while reading a book). By bedtime I was breathing normally. I woke up a couple of times during the night stuffed up, and engaged Alternate Nostril Breathing again. In the morning, after more ginger tea and more breathwork, I felt great, able to facilitate the workshop, and feeling even more impassioned by the power of breath.

"Okay, I'm ready to try," George said with stifled enthusiasm. On the bed, he lay on his right side with his right arm up cradling his head, his mouth closed. I instructed him to plug his bottom (right) nostril with his finger, trying only to breathe out of his upper (left) nostril. After a few seconds he objected. "This is impossible. I can *NOT* breathe! I'm going to suffocate!"

"Just give it some time. Be patient, Love!" I countered. "It'll only take a short time before your sinuses will drain, and you'll be able to breathe out of your upper nostril. Until then use your mouth for teeny bits of air if you really need to."

Within less than ten minutes (time lengthened by additional doubts and distress) he elatedly breathed easily out of one nostril.

"Keep taking deep slow breaths to fully clear it," I encouraged, "and then you can move onto the other side."

After a couple of minutes, George rolled over, repeating the procedure on his left side, allowing his right nostril to clear. With protests lessening, he changed from side to side until both passages remained clear at the same time.

My husband has many admirable qualities, but patience is not always one of them. I hand it to him that he stuck with this for over an hour, albeit between complaints of boredom, monotony, and fatigue, interspersed with exclamations of astonishment that it was really working.

"Okay, now you get to do some real work to make sure the passages stay clear," I optimistically advised him, expecting dispute. To my delight, George felt so surprised he could actually breathe, and perhaps train the next day, that he was inspired to continue. With soothing background music, together we practiced another hour of different styles of Alternate Nostril Breathing that further strengthened the balance he'd achieved by his previous effort.

Breathwork was topped off with soup, ginger tea, and a long soak in a hot bath laced with eucalyptus oil. That night George slept deeply and woke up feeling grand, breathing well through both nostrils. As someone who usually required indisputable facts, or affidavits signed in blood, I hoped he would now see more of breath's merits. I was not to be disappointed.

"It's truly amazing," he commented as he headed out the door for the training, "I never would've believed it."

Was this a one-time thing? If you wonder whether George had to choose between doing what he did for hours, or having access to a drugstore, would he just buy the easier, quicker remedy. It's possible—actually probable that he'd go the faster route—but there are fewer chances for him getting a cold now because he does this breathwork as a daily practice.

Dr. George advises:

One of the most important times to do Alternate Nostril Breathing is when you first wake up. Make sure both passages are clear before you get out of bed. You'll start the day in balance, and it will make a difference.

Although it took years to convince him, George now does it on his own, and we practice various styles together. He often includes Alternate Nostril Breathing in the techniques he imparts for stress management and well-being. Breathing in through your left nostril stimulates the right "feeling" hemisphere of your brain, and breathing in through your right nostril, stimulates the left "thinking" hemisphere of your brain. This breathing allows you to more fully access your whole brain, resulting in better brain functioning, clearer thinking, heightened memory, greater calm, and overall well-being. This breathing is also known to be beneficial in alleviating effects of asthma.

Alternate Nostril Breathing, known in *pranayama* as *nadi shodhana* or *nadi shuddhi*, is progressively showing up in the media with studies that corroborate the benefits.

DEEPENING TIPS: Doctor of yoga and outstanding teacher, Suganya Kumar, instructs that:

"*Nadi* means subtle energy channel and *shuddhi* means cleansing or purifying. This practice cleanses the subtle energy channels so that our prana (life force energy of breath) can flow freely through the body. Inhaling through the left nostril triggers the rest / relaxation response (parasympathetic nervous system) and inhaling through the right stimulates the fight / flight response (sympathetic nervous system).

"By choosing which nostril you use to inhale, you can make yourself either more relaxed (left nostril) or more energized (right nostril). Alternate Nostril Breathing is about bringing these two opposites into balance. By slowly and consciously breathing through each nostril for an equal amount of time, we make sure to stimulate the sympathetic and parasympathetic nervous systems in equal amounts. There are immense health benefits recorded by regular practice of this pranayama. A few are:

- reduced stress and anxiety,
- improved respiratory health / improved cardiovascular health,
- detoxification, and
- better sleep."

For me, Alternate Nostril Breathing is a daily practice and one of the most important techniques I can share. Personally, I find the time spent on this practice to be worth its weight in gold, in how it helps me to self-soothe, focus, center, and balance, think better, and feel better. I have found it essential whenever I am traveling and feel unsettled or nauseous from winding roads, rolling waves, or turbulence in the air. When riding through mountains, I no longer wait to feel queasy to start practicing. For "preventative medicine," I begin to apply techniques at the journey's onset to prevent, or at the very least, mitigate discomfort.

The yogic science of breath, *pranayama*, finds Alternate Nostril Breathing so intricately beneficial that there are multiple methods of performance, with various ratios of inhaling, exhaling, and breath holding. These advanced methods need to be learned with an experienced practitioner. However, one can simply alternate covering each nostril with a finger and breathing for the same number of breaths or period of time, in order to experience powerful benefits.

Basic Alternate Nostril Breathing

TO BEGIN:

In an erect and grounded posture, take your right hand, and curl the middle and index fingers into the palm as the ring and baby fingers press together. (Left hand rests in your lap.) You may reverse these instructions to use your left hand.

Consciously make all inhales and exhales full, gentle, and quiet.

Start by inhaling through both nostrils, and

1. Place your right thumb over your right nostril. From your left nostril exhale and then immediately inhale.
2. Close the left nostril with your ring and baby fingers pressed together.
3. Remove your thumb in order to exhale from your right nostril and then follow with an immediate inhale.

   Going from side to side, repeat for two to ten minutes, or longer.

Dr. George adds:
We know to be in parasympathetic (rest and digest) mode is ideal, and Alternate Nostril BLIPPs take us there. Parasympathetic receptors in our bellies and our noses tell the brain (limbic center) that we are safe. Proactively, daily performing these techniques, especially when stressed, is practicing Breath Literacy at its best.

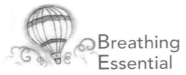

Breathing Essential

Maintaining clear nasal passages is vital to our health and well-being.

BLIPP

Before getting out of bed in the morning, if one nostril is more open than the other, lie on your side with the more plugged nostril on top as you close your bottom nostril with your finger or thumb. Breathe consciously as you take the time for your sinuses to drain until both nostrils remain open.

chapter nineteen

Breathe In Peace / Breathe Out Pain

The Bip / Bop Breath

Please don't think because of its acronym, that this breath is trivial. Quite the contrary, I feel the Bip/Bop Breath (Breathe In Peace/Breathe Out Pain) is one of the most important and powerful breaths to know and utilize. Forget the drum rolls—bring on the full orchestra! This single breath can change your life.

Think of this! We are breathing and thinking all the time but usually without awareness. The act of engaging our prefrontal cortex, executive functions, and power of intention to consciously "Breathe In Peace" in order to let go and "Breathe Out Pain" (whether it be physical or psychological) can begin to change our physiological state. The benefits of the Bip / Bop Breath are phenomenal.

1. We gain more vitality, passion, courage, patience, focus, and peace.
2. We become more relaxed, lighthearted, and laugh easier, catalyzing positive changes for our nervous system and health.

Thus we enhance and empower our lives while bringing more harmony to our relationships, workplaces, and the world at large. What we do with our breath can seem so insignificant, but actually its significance is monumental. *As is the microcosm, so is the macrocosm:* our personal peace leads to planetary peace.

"Imagine."

•   John Lennon   •

In this crazy world we live in, many are not so sure that peace is possible. I get it. I've been there. I have at times witnessed myself sinking to places of deep despair about humanity and our planet. I feel I might be there still if it were not for the Bip/Bop breath and a remarkable Japanese man named Masaji.

When the atomic bomb exploded on Hiroshima, Masaji was fourteen years old, working in a factory outside the city. Reeling from the aftershock of the surreal blast and covered with cuts, one thought alone consumed him: he had to find his family. He took off running in the direction of his home near the epicenter of the explosion, now a living hell. Suddenly surrounded by death, destruction, and unbearable heat, Dante's Inferno had become his reality.

Masaji skirted around people with skin melting off their bones. Those who sought cooling in the river, screamed from the pain of scalding water. Masses of burn victims wailed, moaned, and begged for help. Oblivious to their pleas, his legs propelled him forward as if in a dream. Coming upon his home, Masaji fell to his knees. Before him lay incinerated rubble. Except for a brother away in the army, his entire family had been cremated; his whole world turned upside-down.

After two long years of grief, anger, and desperation, like a phoenix rising out of ashes, Masaji discovered the way to exit his dark night of the soul. He began the practice to very consciously "Breathe In Peace" and "Breathe Out Pain," leaving the past behind.

After learning how to find peace in himself, Masaji then dedicated his life to promoting peace on the entire planet. He spent the next six decades traveling the globe, sharing peace practices through rituals and theatrical productions.

When I first met him in Hiroshima at the Peace Hotel, Masaji was almost seventy, sporting jet-black hair and a huge smile, looking thirty years younger. Although under five feet tall, he loomed a giant of peaceful strength.

Masaji became for me an inspiration in difficult times. He was a living, breathing example that, no matter the depth of misery we might encounter in life, languishing in a place of despair serves no one. He breathed, talked, and "walked the talk" that personal and planetary pursuits of peace must become essential goals for everyone: individuals, groups, and nations.

Dr. George adds:

We know that the chronic stress of constant emotional pain has physiological and mental health consequences. Now we will talk about how chronic stress can adversely impact us on a cellular level and affect how we age.

Within the nucleus of each of trillions of cells in our body we have 23 pairs of chromosomes that contain many of our genes. Our gene codes for all of our characteristics, hair color, height, etc., are organized on a DNA strand. At the ends of these DNA strands are protective caps, similar to the ends of shoelaces, called telomeres. Telomeres help maintain chromosome stability.

According to biologist Dr. Bill Andrews, the average length of a telomere is 15,000 bases at conception. As our cells divide, we lose telomeres. By the time we are born, the telomeres have reduced dramatically to 10,000. Andrews asserts that when telomeres reduce to about 5,000 bases, they lose functionality and that's when a cell dies. This is how we age. Factors accelerating the shortening of telomeres include obesity, smoking, consistent emotional distress, and chronic stress. In other words, when a fight, flight, or freeze response is habitual, telomeres shorten, and aging is accelerated. Short telomeres are associated with cancer, cardiovascular disease, Alzheimer's, and other diseases.

Focusing on positive, peaceful attitudes helps to maintain our telomeres. Anything we can do to mitigate chronic stress and consistent emotional angst helps. These include exercise, proper nutrition, healthy weight, meditation, mindfulness, and of course, breath awareness and BLIPPs, of which the Bip/Bop Breath is excellent.

It doesn't help us to hold on to the past or negativity. The Bip/Bop Breath can be like a computer deleting old files that no longer serve to make room for new "updated software" that does.

"There is no way to peace; peace is the way."
• A. J. Muste •

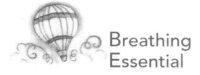

Breathing Essential

With our breath we take in and let go, physically, mentally, emotionally, and spiritually.

BLIPP

Take a walk and set a strong intention to "Bip/Bop." On your exhale, intend to energetically let go of any pain, be it physical, mental, or emotional. On your inhale, breathe in a sense of peace and well-being.

chapter twenty

Feeling on Top of the World

Breathing to Calm, Enjoy, and Empower

Put on a virtual backpack please, as I'd like you to metaphorically join me on a journey to Nepal. As I've shared, I discovered so much about breath while trekking—physical facts of course, but also mental, emotional, and spiritual learning. On my second trip, I was reeling from one of those unforeseen and unwanted experiences that pulls the rug out from under you, bursts your bubble, turns your world upside-down, and literally and figuratively brings you to your knees. I was in such emotional pain, I didn't quite know how to be with myself.

> "Nepal is here to change you,
> Not for you to change Nepal."
> • Sign on trekking post •

Unfortunately (or fortunately) when trekking, you cannot get away from yourself. Unavoidable situations present a crash course on mindfulness; one defining characteristic: being where your feet are. On the trail, you must be where your feet are, grounded in your body, or you could trip, sprain your ankle, fall into oblivion, or be stampeded by donkeys or yaks. If your mind takes you elsewhere, the blisters and throbbing of your feet, the aches in your knees, and the weight of your pack, bring you back. There is no escaping. You have yourself as company, whether welcome or not. And if circumstances are such, pains of the body may be accompanied by pains of the heart.

In the science of yoga, which encompasses every aspect of life, our physical, mental, and emotional bodies interface and affect each other. Emotional pain had cracked my heart open; my shoulders caved in, in protection. Only a scheduled Himalayan trek kept depression from immobilizing me. Had I remained home, I'd have vegetated on my bed or couch, sleeping or numbing myself in any number of ways.

Instead, I arrived in Nepal looking and feeling like a zombie. Luckily no luxury of lethargy was mine. Since I was trekking, I had to get up and move, climbing up or down, eight to fourteen hours a day. Putting one foot in front of the other, with accompanying breath, seemed like an exceptional accomplishment. I could barely muster the effort and while in the loftiest altitudes, I found myself in the lowest plummets of the "roller coaster" of life. *AAAhhhhhhhhhhh!* With the wisdom of hindsight though, I perceive it now as a training ground of extraordinary elevation. That was where and how I discovered the Bip/Bop breath of the previous chapter. It occurred naturally as a way to just keep moving. As I walked, when inhaling, I told myself, *I Breathe in peace.* While exhaling, *I Breathe out pain.* Sometimes the words changed, but the essence remained the same:

I breathe in joy. I let go sorrow.
I breathe in lightness. I breathe out heaviness.
I breathe in love. I let go fear.
I breathe in acceptance. I breathe out disgust.
I breathe in forgiveness. I let go blame.

Of course, I didn't believe it at first, but since it helped me move, I pretended. Breathing out pain and breathing in peace became my mantra even when I slept. I repeated this for hours and hours, hundreds and hundreds of times, with each stride—narrow or wide. Without knowing exactly when, my body/mind started to believe this programming. My breath deepened, life force flowed more fully, my mind calmed, steps became lighter, and my outlook brighter. My posture straightened, and I looked less like the walking dead.

Best-selling author and meditation teacher, Jack Kornfield, inspired by ancient wisdom, wrote: "At the end of the day what matters most is: How fully did you live? How fully did you love? How fully did you let go?"

To these I add: How fully did you breathe?

I had arrived in Nepal energetically weighing a ton. When I departed, the bulk of the burden had been shed along the trails, step by step, breath by breath. In a month, it felt like I'd acheived a year's worth of healing. This is what the breath is about—this beautiful, poignant cycle of taking in and letting go. Just as our respiratory system helps us digest food because of the exchange of gases in the lungs converting food into energy, *our breathing helps us to energetically digest life experiences.* We can store the experiences and learnings that nourish us, and eliminate or let go of the ones that do not.

"If you have never suffered a broken heart,
you will not learn to be truly alive."
• Janie Browen-Whelden •

Please know that whatever heart-wrenching experiences you may have had, or will have (accidents, betrayal, breakups, calamities, crashes, cruelty, death, disease, devastation, destruction, terror, trauma), with your breath and intentions you have abilities to help:

- absorb the good and leave the bad,
- retain the positive and refuse the negative,
- accept a new life trajectory and discard the planned one,
- take lemons and make lemonade, and
- find gifts in the problem—open them—and leave the "wrapping" behind.

It's pretty much impossible to experience life without some heartbreak. Author Curtis Tyrone Jones describes it as: "Some days punch us in the gut so hard, it seems we can feel the whole universe gasp with despair." In these situations, it is empowering to know that we have immediate access to restorative tools. The Bip/Bop of *Breathing in peace and Breathing out pain* can offer healing and empowerment for any type of loss or heartache.

In mindfulness practices, the breath can be an anchor to non-judgmentally become aware of our thoughts—a very worthy and evidence-based, beneficial practice. But what happens when we feel not just hurt, but overwhelmed, devastated, or shattered? How do we manage the experiences of unusual anguish, desolation, and raw pain—be it physical, mental, emotional, or spiritual?

These circumstances require more than mere observation. If we had an open, bleeding wound, we wouldn't just watch it flow. Maintaining our health, well-being, and perhaps our very life itself, requires us to halt the "hemorrhaging."

Intense psychological pain calls for techniques that will change our brains and physiologies rapidly! When possible, we can cry, sob, and maybe even wail. These reactions catalyze deep belly breathing and we know the beneficial results. This is comparable to "flushing out poisons." Now we need a practice that is analogous to applying soothing balm to accelerate healing, or a pump propelling toxic blood out and fresh blood in. Enter the Bip/Bop breath.

Quantum physics tells us that *everything* is vibration. That includes our emotions which vibrate at different frequencies. Some are life-enhancing, and others are life-draining. The life-enhancing emotions/vibrations feel good, and the life-draining ones do not. With our power of free will, we can consciously choose which ones we want to have as part of us and which ones we don't. You can name the feeling, emotion, or experience if you like, or, you can just feel it or visualize it. You can be very detailed, or default to breathing in peace, wellness, and love, and breathing out pain, panic, and fear.

Another way of looking at this practice is that of the Native American sage who tells his grandson about the two wolves living in his heart. He describes the first wolf as angry, mean, fearful, and unhappy, with a tendency toward violence. The other wolf is easygoing, kind, loving, joyful, and focused on peace. The grandfather continues, "At times, they fight with each other." His curious grandson asks, "Who wins?"

The wise elder replies: "The one I feed."

Despite what you may be experiencing, performing the Bip/Bop Breath will begin a clearing to help bring peace and well-being back into your life. An analogy: Think of difficult and painful emotions as a glass of dirty water. If clear water is continually poured into the glass, the sludge must eventually empty out.

DEEPENING TIP: Check out holotropic or transformational breathwork as powerful tools for emotional release. Also, many people find working with Tapping or EFT—Emotional Freedom Techniques (the psychological acupressure techniques that work with the electromagnetic currents running through our bodies) to be highly effective in helping to achieve emotional balance.

BREATHE IN:
peace • calm • love • life • pleasure

BREATHE OUT:
angst • worry • fear • apathy • pain

BREATHE IN:
anticipation • gratitude • trust

BREATHE OUT:
dread • fault-finding • doubt

BREATHE IN:
wonder • acceptance • order

BREATHE OUT:
foreboding • regret • turmoil

BREATHE IN:
simplicity • joy • lightness

BREATHE OUT:
chaos • grief • heaviness

BREATHE IN:
hope • ease • celebration

BREATHE OUT:
despair • effort • lamentation

BREATHE IN:
harmony • timelessness • serenity

BREATHE OUT:
discord • urgency • commotion

BREATHE IN:
abundance • splendor • silence • light

BREATHE OUT:
lack • squalor • uproar • darkness

BREATHE IN:
happiness • grace • forgiveness

BREATHE OUT:
depression • shame • blame

BREATHE IN:
strength • health • well-being

BREATHE OUT:
weakness • illness • misery

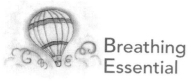

Breathing
Essential

Mind plus emotions, plus breath, acting in unison, equals empowerment.

BLIPP

You may perform the Bip / Bop Breath for others: "May _____ be filled with peace. May _____ be free of pain, etc." Picture and feel the person healthy, happy, and at peace.

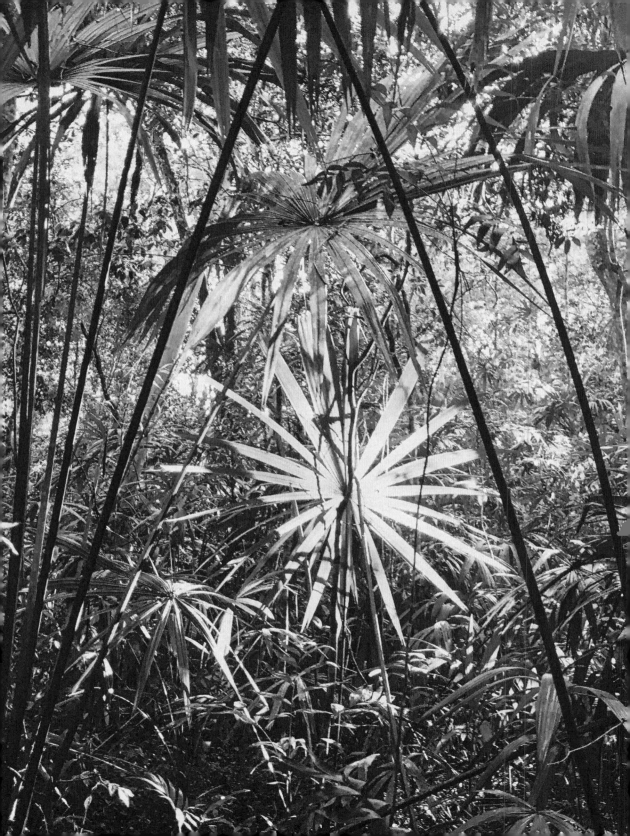

IV

your medicine chest

chapter twenty-one

Take Your Medicine

A Dose of Breath for Health and Well-Being

Yogi Ramacharaka wrote in *The Science of Breath*, "The very simplicity of correct breathing keeps thousands from seriously considering it, while they spend fortunes in seeking health through complicated and expensive procedures and medicines."

Can you imagine a medicine that:

- is always easily accessible?
- is 100 percent organic?
- promotes clear thinking?
- generates serenity?
- energizes the body?
- aids sleep with absolutely no side effects?
- doesn't taste bad nor is hard to swallow?
- is complementary and beneficial to allopathic and holistic treatments?

And (this requires drum rolls, trumpets, and full crescendo):

- costs nothing!

Are you beside yourself with excitement? As you are coming to understand, this isn't just wishful thinking. This "medicine" exists, with curative qualities, and especially preventative powers. This treatment potential is in your every breath. About 400 BC, Hippocrates said, "Let food be thy medicine." He understood that how we nourish our bodies greatly determines the prevention of disease and enhanced well-being. BreathLogic advocates "Let breath be thy medicine."

Consider these definitions of *medicine*:

- *Dictionary.com*: Any substance or substances used in treating disease or illness.
- *Merriam-Webster*: Substance or preparation used in treating disease; something that affects well-being.

The most accessible substance for affecting well-being is the life force flowing in our own breath! We nourish our bodies by how we eat, and likewise we nourish our bodies and entire being by how we breathe.

This is *"maaaaaaaahhh*-velous" news because we're constantly breathing—wherever we are. We aren't required to go anywhere, purchase any equipment, or wear special clothes. Think of all the time, money, and effort we save. We help the environment, consume less, and leave a lighter footprint. We don't have to add another item to our to-do list in order to enhance our well-being. We only have to become aware of something that we're already doing, all of the time, and then make a deliberate change in how we do it.

Yes, it is that simple and that powerful. For centuries, sages in all parts of the world relied on breathing practices for increased well-being and empowerment. *This knowledge used to be kept secret, reserved for the elite, but now it is easily accessible and enhancing lives everywhere.*

Modern science continues to validate what yogic and other Eastern disciplines have understood for more than 4,000 years: the breath, as energy medicine, is significant in every aspect of life. The results of multitudes of studies substantiate that breath awareness and breath practices lead to the healing of stress, emotional problems, and substance abuse, as well as releasing unconscious blocks, fears, and anxieties. Western medicine is beginning to embrace and utilize this knowledge with patients in clinics and hospitals.

The wonder of this "medicine" is that it is already helping prevent maladies that would normally bring people to clinics and hospitals. This is empowering, yet it also necessitates the responsibility of both breathing well and eating well.

For many, this new awareness and practice requires a conscious paradigm shift because it is still so much easier to say, "Just give me a pill or that cold medicine." Nevertheless, a wellness evolution is occurring with optimal breathing at the helm. In areas of the world where there are no hospitals, nor easy access to doctors or drugs, the knowledge of the medicine inherent in our breath can be transformational. James Pearson, an advanced emergency medical technician, (AEMT), relates, "Complaints of SOB (shortness of breath) make up half of our call volume."

Dr. Richard P. Brown, coauthor of *The Healing Breath*, talks about a colleague of his who took a year's sabbatical from the hospital she worked at in New York to treat people in Africa. The caring doctor was looking forward to treating all kinds of exotic illnesses. She was not prepared to have the majority of cases be common stress-related ailments that breathing techniques could help.

When George and I were first living in Colonia Nueva Esperanza (New Hope Village) outside Guatemala City, we witnessed this same phenomenon. It was not dire diseases that mainly affected the residents, but the day-to-day, sometimes moment-by-moment stresses of how to eke out a living. We witnessed how extreme deprivation can take its toll on body, mind, and spirit, how poverty and wealth can be states of mind, and how breath practices can create and support stress resiliency.

Once I had gained their trust, the village women began to come to our home for "yoga." They lived in homes without the ease of running water. In the midst of raising children, making tortillas from scratch, washing clothes by hand, and working from daybreak to bedtime, they seldom took time to nurture themselves. As indigenous women who did not own pants, they came in skirts, which at first threw me for a loop, as I needed to change my lesson plan. Our yoga became fully focused on relaxation, something these women infrequently experienced. The first morning I put on soothing music and led them in exercises in which they slowly, consciously moved their bodies while focusing on their breath.

Upon opening their eyes, their profound reactions surprised and delighted me. Doña Isela, appearing euphoric declared, *"Me sentia en las nubes . . .* I felt like I was in the clouds . . . I have never felt such peace in all my life!"

Sally, a dynamic, passionate advocate for breath, and member of BreathLogic's board, attributes her ability to heal from being hit and disabled by a Mack truck to her breathwork. The initial car accident literally took her breath away and then kept it shallow for a period of two years while she grappled with trauma, anxiety, and inability to fully function, physically and psychologically. It was only when she discovered that her breath held tools that she could consciously harness, that she gratefully related, "I was able to breathe myself back to health, even when I was told I couldn't."

Growing up in Poland in a family with five generations of documented heart issues, my friend, Gosia, related that as a child she was never able to participate in activities with other children. "A few times per day I had tachycardia attacks (about 250 heart beats per minute). Some of these attacks ended with bradycardia and passing out." At age twenty-one (2004) with a diagnosis of vasovagal syndrome, doctors implanted a pacemaker. Although no longer passing out, tiredness, low energy, and arrhythmia were still normal states.

In 2010 Gosia joined her first breathing workshop and started to practice several times per week and often daily. Year by year she began feeling better, more energetic and with less arrhythmia. For the first time she began participating in sports activities without being tired. In her words: "In 2017 I was on holiday in Egypt. I was diving for the first time in my life and I had the same oxygen consumption as my instructor with thirteen years' experience who was diving three to four times per day. He couldn't believe that it was my first dive. He thought that I was diving for many years, just joking with him for fun. After that, I realized that *something big has happened in my life.*"

Gosia asked to have her pacemaker removed. Her doctors were alarmed! They had never experienced removing a pacemaker without implanting another. Finally after heart monitoring determined the pacemaker was truly no longer needed, in 2019 the pacemaker was removed.

"Now, I can say, I am healthy, full of energy, I do fitness, yoga, I am diving and planning a parachute jump. And it all happened because I was doing breathing techniques."

Please be assured that I realize there are reasons and occasions for pills, miracle drugs, and procedures upon which many peoples' lives depend, but when possible, beware of long-term usage that may cause multiple side effects and complications.

As an antidote, remedy, and prescription, long-term daily "doses" of breath practices and routines are a way to "take your medicine"— a medicine that helps prevent dis-ease, and aids in the maintenance and enhancement of your health and well-being. Results may be slower and require personal responsibility, but they are non-toxic, long-lasting, and generally better over time. Breath is medicine we were created with and to which we have constant access.

Andrew Weil MD, wrote in *Breathing: The Master Key to Self-Healing,* "I feel very strongly that proper breathing is a master key to good health. Over and over again, I'm impressed by the power of the breath and its ability to correct specific health problems and promote our general wellness."

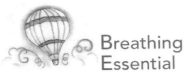

Breathing
Essential

Awareness of your breath and breath practices as daily routines, act as powerful, preventative, and recuperative medicine.

BLIPP

Choose at least one BLIPP or BLIPP routine that you will commit to practicing every day at approximately the same time for an entire year.

chapter twenty-two

The Heart of the Matter

Breath=Heart

According to "The Wise Ones" at Sacsayhuaman, Peru, "It's not so much about who, or where, or why, or how, you are living your life, but rather so much about the amount of love that is expressed at any given moment, moment by moment, breath by breath."

A FABLE

God wanted to hide love from humans. He thought about all the places he could conceal it: in the forest, the sea, a mountain—somewhere very difficult to find. He realized though that humans love to travel and explore, so eventually they would come upon it. With all-knowingness, he grasped that humans always look for love outside themselves—in other people, places, occupations, food, in bars (the chocolate kind and pubs), anywhere but inside themselves.

"Ha ha," God chuckled. "I'll hide love someplace they will never think of looking—their hearts."

A little Zeus-like, God was so delighted with his cleverness that he decided to do the same thing with wisdom. Feeling amused, he thought of how humans seek out clergy, sages, psychics, sacred sites, and search engines, going anywhere but inside themselves. He chortled as he realized, "I'll just hide it alongside love!"

If possible, please put a hand on your heart and notice your breath. Can you sense how your lungs seem to embrace your heart? When we focus on our breath, we automatically engage our hearts—it's an anatomical given. Our lungs physically and energetically encase our hearts.

French physicist and philosopher Pascal believed, "Our hearts have wisdom which wisdom knows not of." Spiritual teacher and author, Adyashanti, explains "Wisdom without love is like having lungs but no air to breathe. Do not seek wisdom in order to acquire knowledge but in order to live and love more fully."

Ahhhhhhhhhhhh, can you sense how conscious breathing is a radical act of self-love, nurturance, and caring? It's like powerful medicine—a love potion! Breathing intentionally and deeply is one of the easiest yet most profound ways to love and nurture ourselves. It is saying *YES!* to life in a language our cells understand and to which they immediately respond. If the axiom is true that we must learn to love ourselves before we can truly love others, this is the practice your loved ones will thank you for doing.

To access a deep source of love and wisdom, we just need to *come home* to ourselves; to *feel,* and *be,* and *breathe* into and with our hearts. This physically strengthens our flesh-and-blood hearts and our entire cardiovascular system. Energetically we cultivate ways to listen to, absorb, and act from the vast wisdom of our hearts. The Heart Breath acts like a vehicle to take us "home."

The Heart Breath

Preparation: Stand or sit with hands in *Namaste* (prayer position) at your heart.

1. Close your eyes and take several breaths, connecting with your heart energy.
2. Inhaling, raise your hands past your face to straight up overhead.
3. Exhaling, let the arms slowly come down outstretched on each side, palms facing down.
4. Inhaling, with palms facing up, raise the arms along the same path on each side, to join palms overhead (body temple position).
5. Exhaling, lower the hands down (in front of your face) into the Namaste position to connect with the heart.

Repeat consciously at least seven times. This breath can be executed for extended periods of time with significant benefits.

Benefits:
- Energetically opens the heart, evoking energies of love and wisdom.
- Exercises and strengthens the arms.
- Opens the chest and expands capacity of the lungs.
- Promotes peacefulness, serenity, and tranquility.
- Strengthens the cyclic energies of giving and receiving.
- Cultivates subtle yet powerful energetic healing of the heart.

Have you ever wondered why most of the world prays with their palms together at the heart—a naturally expressive gesture that is also a salutation in the East and the "Namaste" that ends many yoga classes? Called *Anjali Mudra* in Sanskrit, this hand position means "Salutation Seal."

According to yogic lore, positions of the hands embody great significance. Their physical forms are believed to conduct energy and raise consciousness. Finger and hand positions, called *mudras*, stimulate reflexology pressure points that strengthen body / mind / spirit connections and aid physical, emotional and mental well-being. When left hand fingers (female energy) meet right hand fingers (male energy) to press together at the heart center, this union has balancing effects on the right and left hemispheres of the brain. The mind is calmed, the nervous system soothed, wisdom and love energy of the heart are evoked.

With this mudra, a heart closed and hardened by circumstance, pain, and sorrow can begin to soften and open. The normal chatter of the mind is quieted and one begins to hear the silent sagacity of the heart. A meditative state is achieved and higher consciousness ensues. Performing the Heart Breath, which starts and ends with this mudra, allows us to receive and give, to ourselves and the world, the love energy and wisdom of the heart.

Spiritual teacher, Sai Baba, advises, "It is the heart that reaches the goal; follow the heart." Writer Mark Nepo says it this way: "There is no substitute for following the aliveness that our heart tunes us to." Poet Rumi, inspires us, "Only from the heart can you touch the sky." Doc Childre, founder of HeartMath challenges: "Dare to connect with your heart. You will be lifting not only yourself and those you love and care about, but also the world in which you live."

Dr. George adds:

Let's face it, most of us can be pretty hard-hearted with ourselves. We are often self-critical, with internal dialogues like: *I'm so stupid, how could I have done that? I'm useless, ugly, fat, nobody likes me; I'm not worthy of friendship, respect, or love. I'm not good enough, smart enough, attractive enough, and in reality, there is something seriously wrong with me.*

We can say things to ourselves we would never imagine saying to a friend.

When our sympathetic nervous system triggers emotion—rage, fear, shame—our executive functions disintegrate. In his book, *Emotional Intelligence*, Daniel Goleman calls this "amygdala hijacking." Hijacking some or all of our pre-frontal cortex, taking it offline, can lead to very reactive, defensive, and inappropriate responses. Thankfully, bringing heartfulness and compassion for self and others to these difficult emotional situations can transform how we perceive ourselves or others, and dramatically change how we respond.

Good mental health is positively correlated with higher levels of self-compassion. In their 2017 book, *Handbook of Compassion Science*, Neff and Germer suggest, "Self-compassion is simply compassion directed inward. Just as we can feel compassion for the suffering of others, we can extend compassion toward the self . . . regardless of whether the suffering resulted from external circumstances or our own mistakes, failures, and personal inadequacies."

They describe three components of self-compassion: kindness, common humanity, and mindfulness. Imagine being kind to someone else. Recall the warm feelings associated with reaching out to help and be caring.

Self-kindness is all of that given to ourselves. Daily cultivating an attitude of self-compassion when we are not in a disparaging state strengthens our prefrontal cortex and develops new neural pathways for positive, kind, and compassionate self-talk. Then when actual amygdala hijacking happens, it will be easier to move from berating ourselves to being kind, benefitting us immensely with respect to our mental and physical health, and our interpersonal relationships.

Ahhhhhhhhhhhhhhhhhh. The heart is also connected to the sexual expression of love. Let's change focus a moment to touch on three points of breathing and making love:

1. Making love is so good for the breath; the breath is so good for making love.
2. Better breathing contributes to better sex, foreplay, and afterglow.
3. Whether during sex or just lying together, practice entraining your breathing with your lover's.

My Love,
to feel your heart
beating and breathing
with mine
—sublime
•   LEY   •

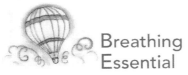

Breathing Essential

When you work with the breath, you automatically work with the heart.

BLIPP

If you have a question or dilemma, sit quietly with a hand on your heart, following your breath. Listen for your heart's wisdom and advice.

chapter twenty-three

Breath Geometry

The Power of the Circle

I invite you now to associate practical geometric shapes with your manner of breathing to improve your breathing skills in ways you can tangibly measure.

Learning geometry is said to help improve logic, problem-solving, and deductive reasoning skills. These abilities are utilized in the living of life itself, but also in art, architecture, engineering, sports, and other disciplines. As the science of geometry helps in the creation of life forms, incorporating basic geometric shapes into the way we breathe can help strengthen and enhance different forms that our lives may take.

We begin our Breath Geometry practice with one of the most ubiquitous forms in nature—the circle. The Circle Breath involves the continuous "taking in of the inhale" and "letting go of the exhale"— each seamlessly merging into the other, equal in length, protective, and unifying. Look around you, wherever you may be, and become aware of all of the circular shapes you see, whether in nature or human-made. Ponder a few moments the symbolism of the circle:

- Never-ending / Connection / Union
- Protection / Fortification / Security
- Equality / Similarity / Impartiality
- Cycles: taking in and letting go, giving and receiving, life-death-rebirth

The significance of the Circle Breath is its smoothness of continual connection without disruption or disturbance; cycles melding easily one into the other.

If you cultivate a daily practice of consciously allowing your breath to be an uninterrupted circle of exhale to inhale, you will soon feel more empowered and "in the flow" with the currents of life. According to mindfulness expert, Jon Kabat-Zinn, "It doesn't have to be for a long time at any one stretch . . . great adventures await you if you give yourself a little time to string moments of awareness together, breath by breath, moment by moment."

So often we hold our breath without even noticing—when we work on our computer, text, read, watch movies, fix meals, etc. We don't even realize it or notice the cycle of tension that is the cause or result. In actual physical danger, this could be a positive "freeze" response, but in normal everyday activity this can weaken our health and well-being. Unconsciously holding out of breath can diminish our vigor, restrict the flow of life, and become an obstacle to feeling fully alive, grounded, and connected to self and others.

Circle Breath Practice

1. Start by watching your breath and simply paying attention to when you are exhaling and when you are inhaling. Notice how one breath flows into the other.
- Notice the physical sensations.
- Observe where you sense movement.
- How does that movement feel?
- Pay attention to yourself paying attention.

2. Witness the natural length of your inhalation. Witness the natural length of your exhalation. Does one feel longer than the other?

- Begin to make them equal by counting in your head the natural duration of your inhale and making your exhale the same length.
- In your practice, whenever it becomes comfortable, increase your breath's length by exhaling for a count longer and then inhaling for a count longer.

Benefits:

- Cultivates mindfulness and calmness.
- Aids in concentration, focus, and patience.
- Slowly, comfortably, begins to increase lung capacity.
- Energizes the body and spirit.
- Enhances overall well-being.

DEEPENING TIP: The importance of going "full circle" is that when we don't breathe in or out, all the way, our diaphragm does not move through the full range of motion with each breath, leaving behind the wrong chemistry of CO_2 and oxygen. This may make us feel anxious, a little out of breath, and off-center.

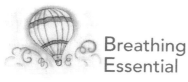

Breathing Essential

Ideally, our breath flows as a river flows—unimpeded.

BLIPP

Close your eyes and allow your breath to circle through your body in even (inhale and exhale) counts for one to ten minutes. As you continue to practice this daily, notice how your count and breath naturally lengthen and deepen.

chapter twenty-four

Long Live the Queen "BE"

Yogic Complete Breath

Ahhhhhhhhhhhhhhh, let go a sigh of relief for a breath so beautiful and sublime—with all of our BLIPPs, we've been preparing for it. But first, let's take a moment to acknowledge how far we have come in integrating the art and science of breath.

- We started naturally to deepen our breath *(simply becoming aware of our inhale and exhale)*.
- We effortlessly deepened the breath more by focusing on *(feeling the physical sensations of the breath)*.
- We began softening away rigidity to naturally awaken the breath and ease our flow of life force *(loosening, bobbing, and shaking)*.
- We supported and strengthened this flow *(assuming excellent posture and grounding (PG))*.
- We utilized the ABC's of Awareness, Balance, and Connection to support our BLIPPs. *(Breath Literacy's Instant Power Practices)*.
- We sighed to let go of tension or increase the benefits of contentment, promoting deeper inhales *(Sighing Breaths)*.

- We've learned to breathe diaphragmatically and be consciously calm while stimulating our parasympathetic nervous system (*Belly / Diaphragmatic Breath*).
- We strengthened the diaphragm and cultivated all the benefits of the Belly Breath, while telling the brain we are safe and happy (*Laughter Practice*).
- We learned to "take In," and "let go" energetically (*Bip / Bop Breath*).
- We've deepened these dynamics through conscious connection of body, mind, and spirit, while opening up the chest (*Heart Breath*).
- We balanced the brain / body systems, increasing abilities to focus, calm, and enhance our overall well-being (*Alternate Nostril Breathing*).
- We strengthened breath awareness and breath flow, cultivating conscious awareness of the cycles in life (*Breath Geometry— the Circle Breath*).

We have slowly and organically been activating our respiratory muscles, expanding our lung capacity, and deepening our body presence to be able to: [Drum roll] *TA DA!* Come to attention in *tadasana* (Mountain Pose) and roll out the red carpet in readiness for "Her Majesty." Imagine hearing a rousing rendition of "All Hail the Queen!"

Enter now, in all her "gradiant" glory, the *Complete Breath*—the queen of breaths!

We have come to a threshold of inviting greater presence and power into our being. We've done the groundwork, and now we've arrived at a ceremonial completion, graduation, and initiation. I say "gradiant" glory because (besides my alliteration fixation) it is a breath that "builds" on itself. Once you establish the Complete Breath as your vital manner of breathing, you will say goodbye, *adios*, and *arrivederci* to respiratory surviving, and be firmly on the royal road to respiratory reviving and thriving.

From childhood, as a form of survival, most us are trained to "buck up" and strengthen our talents to take on and handle more displeasures, disappointments, tasks, and troubles. In a type of misguided machismo, we gained a high range of tolerance for "the difficult." Conversely, most of us would greatly benefit from increasing our abilities to feel good, and welcome more abundance, happiness, freedom, and ease into our lives.

Since *Breath=Life*, if you have been making your unconscious breathing conscious, hopefully you've noticed positive changes spilling over into many areas of life. Now by adding the benefits of the Queen BE—Complete Breath Breathing—we open ourselves to even greater transformation. Instead of continually increasing tolerance for shouldering burdens, challenges, and disappointments, we can begin to lighten our loads. Expanding our lungs organically amplifies our abilities for letting go of problems, and consciously feeling more empowerment, love, joy, and peace. We raise "bliss tolerance" instead of "burden tolerance."

Before I describe the Complete Breath, I want to point out that we have been on a path in this book to which I assign three metaphorical images, from the beginning of our course to where we are now.

VISUAL 1: Imagine a well in a desolate desert. This symbolizes that before realizing that we hold a "well-spring" treasure of resources within, we are barely breathing and completely unconscious of our ordinary breath as a source of extraordinary empowerment.

VISUAL 2: A sprouting desert oasis. Through Breath Literacy and BLIPPs we accept an official "well-come" to begin strengthening our essential life force and "well-being" (puns intended).

VISUAL 3: Now visualize a gorgeous and lush Garden of Eden. We are rocking it with the "Queen BE"—Complete Breath Breathing—enjoying the greatest benefits of any breath so far. We become fully present in utilizing all respiratory muscles and lung cavities, massaging organs of

digestion and elimination, strengthening the heart, more fully oxygen-
ating blood, releasing toxins and enhancing the functioning of all our
body's systems, organs, and glands, while mentally and emotionally
crooning a lullaby to life.

We are more fully, consciously alive with each breath. *Complete
Breath Breathing allows us to smoothly and effectively deepen and lengthen
our breaths to create a state of brain coherence that results in deepest
"well-being"—health, harmony, and homeostasis.*

"Master your breath, let the self be in bliss,
contemplate on the sublime within you."
• T. Krishnamacharya •

The Queen "BE"—The Complete Breath
(Main breath enabling Gosia [page 134] to remove her pacemaker.)

Preparation: Lie down, knees bent if more comfortable, preferably
with one hand on lower belly and the other hand on upper chest.
(This breath may be practiced in any position but lying down is optimal for noticing the physiological effects.)

Relax every part of your body. Breathe steadily in and out
through the nostrils.

3-PART INHALE:

1. Fill the lower belly. (Engage the diaphragm, which exerts a gentle pressure on the abdominal organs, pushing forward the front walls
of the abdomen to expand your lower belly. You may feel this also in
your lower back.)

2. Continue filling the middle belly. (Expand the lower ribs,
breastbone, chest, and middle back.)

3. Fill the upper lungs in the chest. (Expand the rib cage up and out
to the sides as respiratory muscles engage to help move the breath up.)

EXHALE:

4. Like a glass of liquid emptying, exhale slowly and naturally from the top to the bottom of the lungs.

5. Gently contract the muscles of the lower abdomen at the last moment, pressing your navel in toward your spine, so that the following inhale naturally expands the belly.

- Stay focused on *feeling* the physical movement of your breath.
- Inhales and exhales are of equal length.
- As your lung capacity expands and respiratory muscles strengthen, slowly, *comfortably*, begin adding longer counts to lengthen and deepen the breath.

DURATION:

Enjoy for two to twenty minutes, or longer.

DEEPENING TIPS: Upon awakening, in preparation for the day, begin revving up with Belly Breaths and then Complete Breaths. Throughout the day, program yourself to often perform Complete Breaths, whether sitting, standing, or lying down. As preparation for sleep, engage Complete Breaths, first with equal inhales and exhales; then Relaxation Breaths (exhales twice as long as inhales).

The Complete Breath is the fundamental breath of the entire yogic science of breath.

Benefits:
- Brings into play the entire respiratory apparatus, every part of the lungs, every air cell and every respiratory muscle.
- Increases capacity of the lungs.
- Minimum effort leads to maximum amount of benefits.
- Decreases susceptibility to pulmonary and bronchial ailments.

- Increased oxygen resists germs and boosts immune system.
- Improves blood quality / regulates blood pressure.
- Stimulates metabolism / promotes better digestion and elimination.
- Strengthens reproductive functions.
- Encourages restful and rejuvenating sleep.
- Massages, exercises, and tones internal organs, boosting their functions.
- Harmonizes body, mind, and spirit.
- Fosters relaxation / creates stress resiliency.
- Causes calmness, serenity, and peacefulness to become prolonged states of being.

You can now combine practice of the "Queen BE" with Circle Breaths at whatever ratio is comfortable for you. You may find very quickly that you are able to increase your count. *The key is to always remain in the comfort zone and stay relaxed.* Explore the heightened benefits of applying Complete Breath Breathing to BLIPP techniques including Sighing, Bip / Bop Breath, Heart Breath, Alternate Nostril Breathing, and Relaxation Breath.

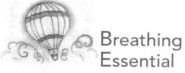

Breathing Essential

Acquiring the ability to perform the Complete Breath is deepening your commitment to yourself and life's potential within you.

BLIPP

Perform Complete Breath Breathing in any position. Feel the expansion of the inhale and the letting go of the exhale in both the front and back of your body.

chapter twenty-five

Pausitive Breath Geometry

The Power of Rectangles, Triangles, and Squares

Very simply and powerfully, the more conscious and comfortable we become with the cycles of our breath, the more conscious and comfortable we become in the cycles of our lives. We flow as our breath flows.

With the Circle Breath as a foundation, we now begin to add conscious breath holding times after the inhale and after the exhale. This "holding" teaches us to become more *pausitive* and experience the benefits of *pausitivity*. Although these words are not in the dictionary *yet*, they precisely describe our next lesson in Breath Geometry. With the Circle Breath, we experience seamless connection between exhales and inhales. With linear breaths, we very intentionally add conscious pauses. We do this for both physical and energetic purposes.

Geometrically, by utilizing four lines or energies, rectangles (a square is a rectangle) are powerful foundational symbols. With resilient stability, they serve as a base to build upon and lend their form to the creation of countless patterns and designs. We often witness the powerful symbolism of "four" in nature:

- Four seasons: spring, summer, fall, winter
- Four directions: north, south, east, west
- Four elements: earth, air, fire, water
- Four cosmic elements: sun, moon, planets, stars

These breaths are best performed with knowledge and application of the Complete Breath in order to most proficiently increase the capacity of the lungs. However, with low counts and only Belly Breaths, virtually anyone can begin practicing them and experiencing their powerful benefits.

CAUTION: If you have respiratory, cardiovascular, or anxiety issues please refrain from engaging in any forms of breath-holding until you check with your doctor. *ALWAYS remain in low, fully comfortable counts.* (Higher counts require a qualified teacher of pranayama, knowledgeable in utilization of bandhas/locks.) If you feel an affinity for these breaths please find a qualified teacher to aid your progress.

Rectangle Breaths

Rectangle Breaths (four-part breaths) are the Circle Breath made linear by adding pauses. We hold full of breath after inhaling, and we hold empty of breath after exhaling. English poet Laurence Binyon wrote, "We too should make ourselves empty, that the great soul of the universe may feed us with its breath."

We begin breathing in the shape of a *tall Rectangle* by inhaling and exhaling twice as long as the times we hold in and hold out. For example, 4-2-4-2: Inhale for 4 counts, hold full for 2. Exhale for 4 counts, hold out for 2. (6-3-6-3 etc.)

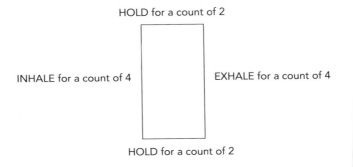

HOLD for a count of 2

INHALE for a count of 4   EXHALE for a count of 4

HOLD for a count of 2

We can also breathe in the shape of a *wide rectangle*. For example, 2-4-2-4: Inhale for 2 counts, hold full for 4. Exhale for 2 counts and hold out for 4. With comfort and practice you can increase the counts to 3-6-3-6, 4-8-4-8, etc.

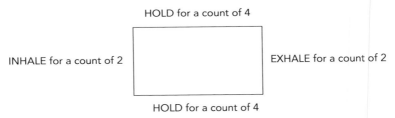

HOLD for a count of 4

INHALE for a count of 2   EXHALE for a count of 2

HOLD for a count of 4

For the rectangle that is the *Square Breath* all lengths are the same. When you practice this breath start with a low, very comfortable count and slowly by one count at a time, build your ability to be present and thus increase all benefits.

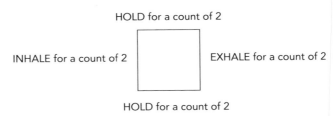

HOLD for a count of 2

INHALE for a count of 2   EXHALE for a count of 2

HOLD for a count of 2

*"Inhale, and God approaches you.
Hold the inhalation, and God remains with you.
Exhale, and you approach God.
Hold the exhalation, and surrender to God."*
• T. Krishnamacharya •

The Square Breath, with inhaling, exhaling, holding in and holding out for four counts each, has been adopted by the U.S. Navy Seals as their "Box Breath." This elite unit must learn to hold their breath for two minutes and the Square (Box) Breath is an important tool for helping them achieve this. Police forces in many areas of the world are also employing "Breath Geometry" in their training. One of my teachers touted these breaths as being very beneficial for aiding heart rate variability (HRV).

Physiological and Energetic Benefits of Pausitive Breath Geometry

INHALE: The deeper and more fully we are able to comfortably inhale and take life force into our bodies, the more:

- oxygen bathes our cells, strengthening, repairing, rejuvenating,
- our muscles of respiration are exercised,
- the quality of blood improves,
- the immune system is enhanced,
- we combat depression, and
- we are able say "yes" to more fully experiencing life.

HOLDING AFTER INHALE: The more consciously and comfortably we are able to be with holding our breath full after inhaling, the more:

- benefits of the inhale are increased,
- the "elasticity" of lung tissues stretches to expand lung capacity,
- the cardiovascular system is strengthened,
- oxygen has the ability to resist germs,

- we foster body presence and grounding,
- we promote harmony between body, mind, and spirit,
- we are able to connect with our heart's desires on a deeper level, and
- we are able to be with fullness, "raising our bliss tolerance."

EXHALE: The deeper and more fully we are able to comfortably empty breath from our bodies, the more:

- we rid ourselves not just of toxins and carbon dioxide but of mental and emotional "debris" that drains our life force,
- our nervous system is soothed,
- our liver, stomach, heart, and other organs are massaged and aided,
- our metabolism is upgraded,
- our blood pressure regulates,
- we relax, and
- we let go of what energetically does not serve us.

HOLDING AFTER EXHALE: The more consciously and comfortably we are able to be with holding our breath empty after exhaling, the more:

- our organs of digestion and elimination are stimulated,
- our reproductive system becomes revitalized,
- we become more stress resilient,
- concentration is improved,
- we cultivate the benefits of silence, stillness, and pause, and
- we are able to learn to trust on a deep, energetic, and spiritual level.

A very significant teacher of mine compared this type of breathing to experiencing in one full cycle of breath, the cycle of the four seasons:

- Inhaling is analogous to spring; saying "yes" to life and rebirth; savoring growth and newness.
- Holding full of breath is like midsummer and basking in the fullness of life; soaking up the sun and the wonders of existence with ease and heartfelt gratitude; revealing our heart's wisdom.
- Exhaling is like a glorious autumn; letting go of what has fulfilled or "fed" us but now has no purpose.
- Holding empty of air is like the starkness of winter; the energy of hibernation, pause, and silent gestation in the womb.

This teacher, who spent winters in the north, explained it this way: "When at the end of May, snow still covers the ground, we'd lose hope of spring except that we absolutely know that every year it comes! It may be late, but it comes. We trust, because that knowing is a part of who we are."

It's the same with the holding out of breath. The more conscious, comfortable, and proficient we can become, the more we incorporate into ourselves the ability to trust—to be in the void. This is so significant! Our bodies and our beings know absolutely that we will breathe again. We can utilize this cycle to help us be calm, peaceful, and trusting while in the unknown, in whichever ways the unknown manifests in our lives. With these practices, we can maintain our equilibrium fostering balance and homeostasis in the cycles of life and health.

"Controlling the volume, duration and frequency
of the inhalation, the exhalation, and the pauses
between each breath enhances prana,
the energy that supports and sustains the life force.
Breathing becomes slow and refined."
- Yoga Sutra 2.50 -

Triangle Breaths

Three-part breaths are a wonderful way to learn breath control, cultivate presence, and increase the capacity of the lungs. They can accentuate the benefits of holding full of breath, or holding empty of breath.

For example, inhale for 2 (or more) counts, hold in for the same count and exhale for the same count. Or inhale for 2 (or more) counts, exhale for the same count and hold out for the same count.

There are many ratios for breathwork. Another example of a 3-part breath: Inhale for 2 counts, hold for 4, and exhale for 3. With a deepening capacity this can quickly become: Inhale for 4 counts, hold for 8 counts, and exhale for 6 counts. A gentle reminder to always stay in your comfort zone.

The effects of these breaths can be described as *pausitively zenulating* or *zenulatingly pausitive*. To me these "words" convey both the peaceful stimulation and invigorating serenity one feels from their forms and spaciousness. I hope that in this chapter you have sensed a systematic, sacred symmetry that will expand your appreciation for the capacity of "pausitive Breath Geometry" to sculpt not just your breath, but also your life.

"Breath being the secret of all being, is the most important of all things."
• Sufi saying •

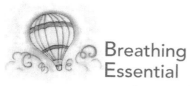

Breathing
Essential

Consciously holding the breath after inhaling and also after exhaling can produce profound physical and energetic benefits.

BLIPP

Develop a habit of performing one to ten Rectangle Breaths and then one to ten Square Breaths before eating a meal.

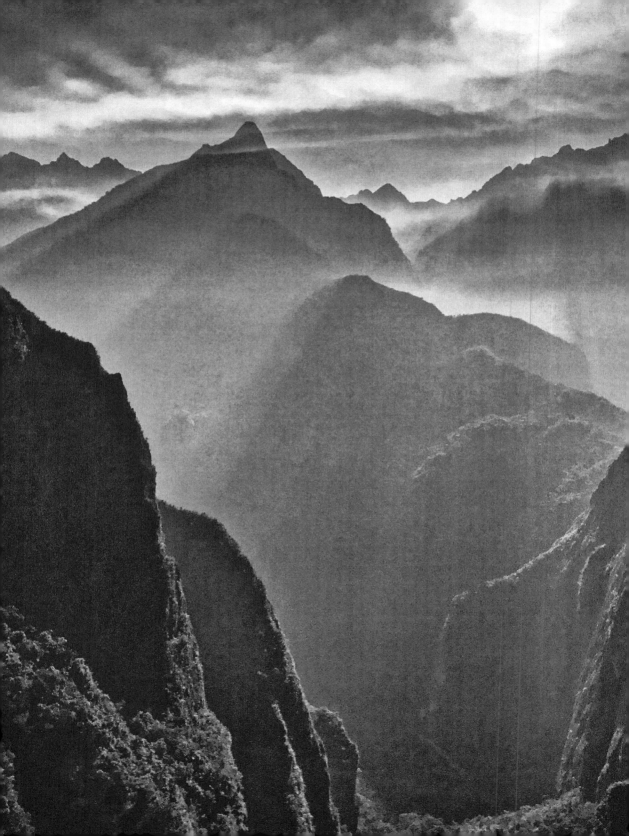

part two

putting understanding
into practice

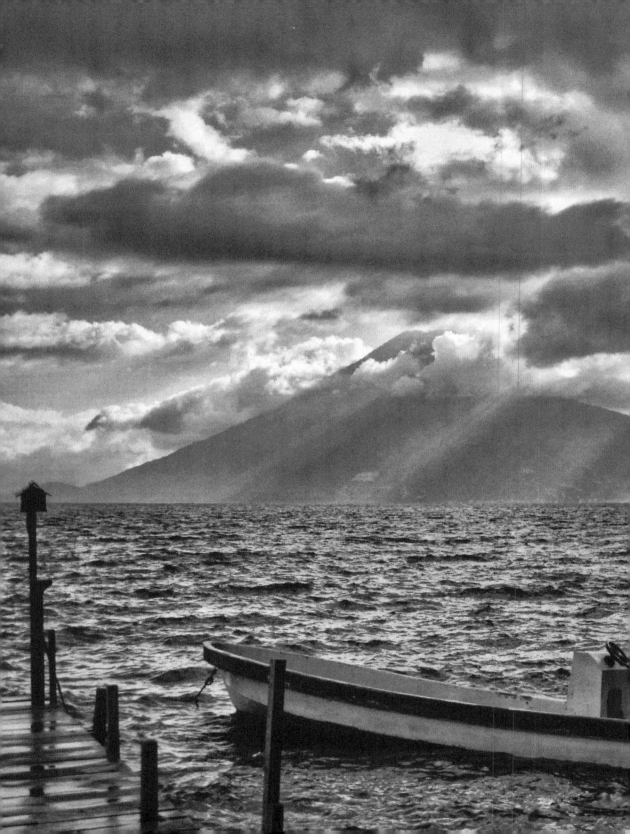

V

the right breath at the right time

chapter twenty-six

Not Just for Beauty

Sleep Is All-Important

*"We can get by on just a few hours of sleep a night.
However, we do nap twelve hours during the day."*
• Ubu, Kukla, and Scheherazade (cats) •

Adequate sleep is essential for well-being, yet sleep deprivation is in the news—a lot! Not just adults, but teenagers and children are also drastically sleep-deprived. This is not good news. It's analogous to learning that millions of people are starving or at the very least deficient in proper nourishment.

Lack of adequate sleep is so common that people just take for granted that "that's the way it is." The Geneva Convention banned sleep deprivation as illegal torture, but it remains something we do to ourselves. Is this not crazy?

People who haven't slept well often look older than those who are rested. They may exhibit dark circles under their eyes, fatigued posture, disheveled hairdos, and pajamas disguised as street clothes.

These visual effects are only the "the tip of the iceberg." Not so apparent, but on the scale of "significant to dangerous," is how lack of sleep affects us throughout our entire being. Our brains cannot function optimally—so every organ, gland, and system in the body reacts by not functioning optimally either. Our cognitive abilities, executive functions, memories, metabolisms, digestive systems, immune systems, and the body's ability to regenerate and rejuvenate are all adversely impacted by not enough Z's.

And as if this isn't enough, we become more accident-prone. Sleep deprivation has been linked to thousands of automobile accidents every year, millions of disability injuries, the catastrophes of the Exxon *Valdez*, space shuttle *Challenger*, Chernobyl disaster, and the Three Mile Island accident. Let's not even mention medical errors.

Experts state that sleeping pills, known to have oodles of injurious side effects, will sedate but do not provide electric readouts that show the brain is performing the important functions that authentic sleep entails. According to sleep scientist Matt Walker, a professor of neuroscience and psychology at the University of California, Berkeley, and author of the book, *Why We Sleep*, "The quality of sleep that you have when you're on these drugs is not the same as normal, naturalistic sleep."

We need sleep like we need to eat and breathe. We are nourished and replenished by the profound relaxation a deep sleep provides. There's not a part of our being that doesn't improve when we have a good sleep: energy level, mood, memory, patience, decision-making, creativity, work, sports, everything! When we haven't slept well, we are not at our best.

With this in mind, think of children and teenagers you may know and love—even ones you don't love. If they're displaying mood swings and aren't acting lovable, perhaps it's because they haven't had enough sleep. Besides being a temperament aid, sleep is fundamentally vital to development during youth and puberty.

Experts say toddlers need about thirteen hours of sleep and naps; around nine-and-a-half hours are needed for teens. Many parents say: "Good luck with that!" Late nights with early school start times interfere with natural circadian rhythms. Stresses of peer pressure, academic demands, and excessive expectations compound to make nine to ten hours of sleep time seem like a daydream at best. Studies relate inadequate sleep to lowered academic performance, depression, child obesity, emotional reactivity, and hyperactivity sometimes misdiagnosed as ADHD. Research shows that many adults have been experiencing the repercussions of insufficient sleep since childhood, with those who sleep under five hours a night having 50 percent more likelihood of obesity. We are usually more stressed if we are tired, and we already know the trajectory that can put us on.

So how can we tell how many hours we need? Eight hours for adults seems to be the number most researchers come up with. However, what does your body/mind want? Some experts say quality of shut-eye is more important than quantity. Do you wake up to an alarm, or do you naturally awaken? Ideally if you can wake up naturally, it is more likely you've received an optimal amount of sleep. However, not everyone has this luxury.

If you must wake up to an artificial device, by all means choose a welcoming sound that invites you to the day. Bringing our consciousness into the morning by the brutal blare or buzz of an alarm sets us up for stress. Think of it! Synonyms for alarm are apprehension, terror, fright, panic, anxiety, distress, and dread. How we transition from the sleep state is extremely important for setting the tone of the day and for our overall well-being.

> "There is no hope for a civilization that starts each day
> to the sound of an alarm clock."
> • Author Unknown •

The quality of our day is affected by how we breathe as we enter into it. If startled by an alarm, we start the day primed for fight, flight, or freeze, breathing shallowly, or holding our breath. Taking the time in the morning to breathe deeply and begin calmly moving *prana* throughout our being in an attitude of gratitude for being alive, primes us to experience the miracles and magic of a new day.

Upon awakening, gift yourself the time to consciously breathe in the qualities you desire to bring into your day. In fact, the manner in which we enter and exit a sleep state can be crucial for our health and balance on all levels. Imagine these various nighttime scenarios:

Scenario 1: Watch TV (horror show, violent drama, the news).
Scenario 2: Text, tweet, upload, download, reload.
Scenario 3: Experience dimmed lights, soft music, hot bath with lavender.
Scenario 4: Raid refrigerator, eat all leftovers, drink alcohol—lots of it.
Scenario 5: Don't eat after dinner, or have a light snack, sip chamomile tea.
Scenario 6: Agonize over the past, fret about the future.
Scenario 7: Focus on following your breath—low and slow, relax, let go.

The scenarios conducive to better sleep are quite obvious, yet although we want to sleep better, we often still indulge. Getting overly stimulated, eating big meals, drinking too much, using technology, and worrying right before bed do not usually contribute to a good night's sleep—or popping out of bed like toast in the morning. What is on our minds when we fall asleep has important bearing on how well we sleep, how rested and revitalized we feel when we awaken, and how well the endocrine system is able to repair our cells as we repose.

Let what you have on your mind be the awareness of your breath, and reap benefits! Focusing on the physical movement of your exhalations as you drift off, and your inhalations when you first awaken, will help breathe calmness into your sleep, vitality into your day, and beauty into your face.

> "When you awake in the morning,
> think of what a precious privilege it is
> to be alive, to breathe, to think, to enjoy, to love."
> •   Marcus Aurelius   •

Be alive!   Breathe!   Think!   Enjoy!   Love!

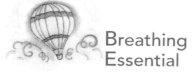

Breathing Essential

The way we breathe when we first come into consciousness helps determine our day. The way we breathe as we retire in bed helps determine the quality of our sleep.

BLIPP

Before getting out of bed in the morning, spend at least five minutes breathing deeply and fully into all parts of your body to bring full presence into your BEing. Practice going to sleep breathing conscious relaxation into every part of your body.

chapter twenty-seven

Now I Lay Me Down to Sleep

When You Can't Sleep

Sleep is so significant for our well-being that it merits another chapter. Comedian W.C. Fields advised, "The best cure for insomnia is to get a lot of sleep." It would be an ideal world if we could do just that! So what do we do when we just can't get to sleep, wake up in the wee hours, work graveyard and erratic shifts, or feel jet lagged?

Whether or not you traverse time zones, consistent sleep deprivation is similar to constant low-level jet lag. Many adults and children experience these symptoms on a regular basis without leaving their homes. According to Harvard neurologist and sleep medicine physician Josna Adusumilli, "Most of us are operating at suboptimal levels basically always. Fifty to seventy million Americans have chronic sleep disorders."

In almost every school where I've engaged students in just ten minutes of closed-eyes relaxation, some little munchkin falls asleep. It's the same with adults. Our bodies and minds crave the restorative benefits of sleep and will grasp the opportunity to avail this natural yearning, nay, requirement. Better to succumb in a controlled environment than a speeding car.

Having lived in time zones eight to twelve hours different from where I often need to be, and never prone to taking sleeping pills, I've become profoundly aware of sleep deprivation's detriments and dangers, along with insomnia's insufferable insanities. That may sound exaggerated, but think about it. There must have been occasions in the last year, month, or week, when you needed to rise early to be present or productive, yet for whatever reason: restlessness, worry, sleeping companion, jet lag, noises, etc., you couldn't sleep. It can make you feel crazy.

Author Jules Verne wrote, "Though sleep is called our best friend, it is a friend who often keeps us waiting!" The latest stats suggest that one out of every three adults experiences insomnia. Sometimes I'm one of them. However, I know a natural solution that is ancient, doesn't cost a cent, and is available to everyone. I've found it to be a life saver. I will tell you up front that it may or may not put you to sleep, but it will help you feel rested as if you've slept. Soundly even! You won't be surprised to know that it has to do with breathing—but how?

Breath and presence! We already know that our breath bequeaths us the gifts of presence. Don't even bother counting sheep, it's your breaths that call out to be counted. This is the time to fully engage the Relaxation Breath (taking the natural, comfortable count of your inhalation and doubling the count for your exhalation) while performing the Complete Breath. For example, inhaling to a count of three, gently expanding your belly, middle and upper chest, then exhaling to a count of six as you consciously, and more slowly, let go. Whenever it feels comfortable, begin lengthening your counts.

With these combined breaths, the PNS becomes dominant. The limbic system of the brain that is wired to find danger lurking, even when and where danger is not, becomes calmed. (Sounds of a burglar are really the house settling.) The longer, languid letting-go of the exhalations takes us deeper into repose. This way of breathing helps us fall asleep and sleep deeper. In the case of jet lag where your body clock won't flip, reposing in this way will, at a minimum, help you feel rested and revitalized.

The most frequent comments I hear from practitioners of this breath are: "I've never slept so well in all my life!" or "I slept like a baby!" or "Were there sleeping pills in the tea?" No, the breath works its own magic. This practice and the ensuing effects of deepening relaxation throughout the body/mind create a type of *yoga nidra*—a state of consciousness between sleeping and waking. This level of profound tranquility that slows our brainwaves to alpha or theta, can provide the sense of energy restoration, regeneration, and rebalancing of actual sleep.

If you can't sleep, learning how your breath can help you to access this state and still receive sleep's benefits will make significant changes in your life. Acquiring this ability to readily relax deeply takes practice. As your mind learns to "chill out" by creating new neural pathways, you can drop the counting, relishing the peace as you focus on the feeling of your exhale letting go and taking you deeper and deeper into presence, repose, and restoration. Try comfortably adding Breath Geometry discussed in chapters 23 and 25 to help you relax even deeper.

Utilizing the mind to tune into the body is the key. At first it may be challenging to hold your focus. With patience and practice, you deepen the neural pathways in your brain that stimulate parasympathetic activity to more quickly take you to relaxation, repose, and regeneration.

DEEPENING TIP: Performing a body scan as you breathe low and slow is proven to be beneficial in deepening relaxation and promoting sleep. Begin at the toes or the top of the head and progress slowly through your body, either up or down, gradually acknowledging, breathing into, and relaxing each body part. Even if you don't fall asleep, the anxiety of not sleeping can be replaced by the assurance that your body/mind will experience replenishment of deep meditation.

Dr. George adds:

There are mainly two types of sleep: non-rapid eye movement (NREM) and rapid eye movement (REM) in four stages of sleep. Stages 1 to 3 are NREM and the fourth stage is REM. There are normally four to five sleep cycles per night; a complete sleep cycle lasting about ninety minutes.

Stage 1—The beginning of the sleep cycle is quite light and considered a transition period between being awake and sleeping. Lasting around five to ten minutes, if awoken during this stage, one might not even realize they were asleep.

Stage 2—This sleep stage lasts longer with decreases in body temperature and heart rate. People spend between forty to fifty percent of their sleep in this stage.

Stage 3—The deepest and most restorative stage of sleep. Muscles are profoundly relaxed with reduction in blood pressure and in respiration.

Stage 4—Rapid eye movement (REM) sleep is known as the dream stage. This stage is characterized as a less-deep sleep. The brain is more active, which is observed overtly through eye movements usually going rapidly back and forth.

These stages are not linear or exactly sequential.

The amygdala (neuroception) is activated when we experience sleep deprivation. The more REM sleep we get, the less reactive our amygdala. No wonder we can trigger easily without adequate sleep.

Suggestions for sleep improvement
• Eliminate or substantially reduce light stimulation for about one hour prior to going to sleep. Sleep in as dark a room as possible or with an eye shade.

- Establish a consistent bedtime.
- Utilize relaxing behaviors to train your brain for sleep, e.g., hot bath, breathing techniques, meditation, peaceful music.
- Train your mind to have positive, gentle, and caring thoughts. These thoughts will tell the amygdala that you are safe (self-soothing). Negative, angry, scared, or worried thoughts will activate the sympathetic nervous system, which is contraindicated for a good sleep. Fight or flight, and sleep are not compatible bedfellows.
- Listen to audio selections related to relaxation and peaceful imagery and ideas.
- Exercise daily.

"True silence is the rest of the mind,
and is to the spirit what sleep is to the body,
nourishment and refreshment."
•   William Penn   •

A strange but lovable dog wandered into a woman's yard one day. She petted him, and he followed her into the house, curled up in a corner and fell asleep. When he awoke, after stretching and shaking, he went to the door to be let out. The next day he came back and again went to what was to become his corner, and took a nap. This routine continued for days. The woman was a little confused. The dog was wearing a collar and appeared well fed and well taken care of, so she could not understand why he was choosing her home to sleep in every day. After weeks of this consistent behavior, she decided to attach a note to the dog's collar: "I would like to find out who the owner of this wonderful sweet dog is," she wrote, "and ask if you are aware that he comes to my house for naps."

She was very curious to find out if there would be a response. Sure enough, when the nap-seeking pet arrived the next day, there was a different note attached to his collar: "He lives in a home with six children, two under the age of three. He's trying to catch up on his sleep. Can I come with him tomorrow?"

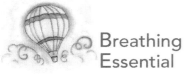

Breathing Essential

If you cannot sleep, use your breath to help you create a relaxed state.

BLIPP

Focus awareness on the Relaxation Breath, exhaling twice as long as your inhalation. As you exhale, intend deep surrender and letting go.

chapter twenty-eight

ABC's of Performance

Breathing for Empowerment

In my first yoga teacher training, the head instructor informed us that there was only one rule for our style of Hatha yoga: *non-competition*. At least with others. It did not matter what anyone else could do. The goal was to let our own bodies guide us deeper into poses without force. Not mind *over* matter—mind *with* matter. We were advised, "Find your edge; be with it, breathe with it. Respect your edge as the wisdom of your body that protects you from injury. Don't force. Let your breath show you when you are ready. Allow this connection of body, mind, and spirit to be what empowers your practice."

Not all yoga styles are like this, and nor are most sports. Pushing oneself is the established path to improvement, yet breath still plays a major role. Whether for personal enjoyment or professional sports competition, practitioners can enhance their skills with the "ABC's of Breath Literacy" from chapter 11. For this chapter, we rename them the "ABC's of Performance." They're still the same: Awareness, Balance, and Connection, but let's look at them through the lens of implementing performance prowess.

AWARENESS: Become aware of your body in regard to the space around you—proprioception, which utilizes sensory feedback mechanisms for motor control and posture. To practice:
- Utilize the breath to consciously and fully inhabit your body. (This awareness aids muscle contraction required as immediate response to incoming information from outside stimuli.)
- Notice where your feet are in regard to your neck and head. (This strengthens full-body awareness.)

BALANCE: Become grounded and centered in your being. To practice:
- "Plant" your feet (toes included) to establish them as a foundation.
- Feel your weight balanced in your torso and centered between front-to-back and side-to-side. Knees are relaxed. (Let movements come from this place of solidity and empowerment.)

CONNECTION: To practice:
- Become deeply aware (mind), of the physical feeling (body), of your breath flowing (spirit) in your belly/core (empowerment).
- Breathe with awareness of being supported by the Earth and heavens (an ancient method native peoples have utilized to experience additional sources of energy and empowerment).

The goal is to consciously practice these ABC's so that they automatically become part of who you are. In some sports, these adjustments are the foundational send-off for the entire activity. In others, the performer comes "home" to them repeatedly. Ideally these ABC's reset "calibrations" (sometimes thought of as muscle memory) without thinking. You can observe this in all ball players, golfers, skaters, weightlifters, and other athletes.

To enhance performance skills, it is crucial to develop a foundation of breath work that supports and augments personal workout programs. The value of this groundwork cannot be overemphasized:

- Breathe through your nose whenever possible. (Exhaling through the mouth is often acceptable. During short intensive periods, one may breathe in and out through the mouth).
- Practice bouncing or shaking to rev up your lymph system, loosen rigidity, and get the breath flowing. (chapter 13)
- Become adept at Diaphragmatic/Belly Breathing. (chapters 14 and 15)
- Practice deepening and lengthening your breath by utilizing:
  Alternate Nostril Breathing
  Relaxation Breaths
  Kapalabhati/Fire Breaths (visit www.BreathLogic.org)
- Become skilled in Complete Breath Breathing and intensify this mastery with Breath Geometry. (chapters 23 and 25)

Many high-performing athletes improve their skills by enhancing their breathing—from Navy SEALS to mountain climbers, to ironmen, to free divers, among others. The amount of improvement depends on how much they have already developed their breath.

Special Operations (Navy SEAL) Senior Chief Petty Officer Sheldon J.S. relates:

"Several years ago, my wife and I participated in Laurie's Power of Breath workshop. I wasn't skeptical but was somewhat hesitant to see if this was the right venue to learn and apply calming techniques. After the class was over, I knew I could turn to these learned tools for the rest of my life and use them during work and deployments. I have since used breathing techniques to improve both my personal and professional life. More importantly, I have passed this knowledge on to other SEAL teammates and many students by showing them the effectiveness of Diaphragmatic Breathing and how to truly harness the power of one's breath. There are many examples where I have incorporated this into training and work:

- 'Focused breathing' was included in curriculum to aid in mid to long range target accuracy . . . for clarity and settling heart rate.
- Using breath control and Diaphragmatic Breathing was tremendously beneficial while on combat diving training evolutions, allowing more air to stay in the oxygen tank and keeping us more relaxed throughout the entire dive.
- While deployed, deep breathing helped to calm nerves, remain focused and confident in all phases while planning for and being on combat missions. For me . . . specifically sitting on a helicopter is where I'm the most anxious, although by keeping my eyes closed, breathing very deeply through my belly had a 100 percent calming effect on my entire mind and body.
- Post missions, turning off a heightened nervous system can be challenging, though adapting focused breathing significantly helped reduce my stress and mitigate anxiety. Additionally, this helped to get to a state of rest easier, and allowed sleep without turning to sleeping pills."

Michael, a Red Sea free diver, after only one session focusing on acquiring Complete Breaths and Breath Geometry, was quickly able to increase his breath-holding time by a full minute.

After working with these breaths in high altitude in Peru, a triathlete, Ron, exceeded his performance expectations in a Colorado triathlon and then in an Ironman competition in Minnesota. He reports: "Initially I was interested in improving my L.D. (long distance) running. Techniques from Laurie's classes enhanced my running later in five Pikes Peak Marathons, a hundred mile, Himalayan-five-day stage race in the foothills of K2 (Mt. Kangchenjunga), India, and an ultra-marathon of fifty miles."

These breathing techniques are not mine, they are universal. What I've done in teaching countless Power of Breath workshops is to hone the practices and the way they are taught. I discovered it is important to bypass the judgment of the mind that tends to tell us we're doing something wrong. Thus we focus first on cultivating nonjudgmental, nurturing presence, and then later work with the "mechanical correctness" of the techniques. Learners do not "get" the practices from only their minds: rather, they learn holistically; bodies, minds, and spirits together. How well a person is able to "inhabit" their body will determine the speed at which they can integrate practices. The beauty of the breath is that, although a personal trainer may be ideal, if disciplined on your own, you can accomplish more than you may ever have dreamed possible. To remind and underscore:

It is necessary first of all to:
1. Become conscious of your breathing, *feeling* your breath.
2. Master the Diaphragmatic/Belly Breath and Complete Breath.
3. Incorporate the Breathing Essentials into your way of Being.
4. Cultivate BLIPPs (Breath Literacy's Instant Power Practices) as a way of life.

Star athlete, Shaquille O'Neal, affirms, "Excellence is not a singular act, but a habit. You are what you do repeatedly." Yoga teacher and sports breathing specialist, Jessica Owens, reminds us, "For all sports, it is important to breathe deeply rather than take shallow breaths. To breathe deeply, you should feel the breath originate in your low abdomen, your diaphragm lift, and your lungs expand. Breathing deeply oxygenates your muscles so they can work harder, build strength, and move faster. After you learn to breathe deeply, the challenge is to feel comfortable with the breathing rhythm that is optimal for the sport you are doing, whether it's running, swimming, yoga, or any other physical activity."

Do you want to know who else will surely benefit from breath awareness and practices during stressful competitive events? Whether watching live or armchair, the loved ones and fans rooting in the audience may be the "anxiously breathing or non-breathing supporters." Whether viewing the Olympics, or kid's soccer, spectators can also benefit from applying the ABC's of Performance.

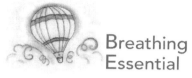

Breathing Essential

The ayurvedic approach to exercise suggests nose breathing instead of mouth breathing during exercise to replace exercise stress with a chemistry of composure and calm.

BLIPP

While walking, running, biking, other sports—practice synchronizing the Rectangle Breath and Square Breath to your movements.

chapter twenty-nine

Being a "Good Sport"

Breathing and Winning

I'd like to tell you about the most amazing sports person I've person-ally met. This woman is extraordinarily inspirational in how she has used breath in athleticism and in life. An award-winning athlete, she has broken world records—in distance and sprinting—in national and international events, and holds a record that can never be broken.

The young Lindsay Nielsen reminds me of a character from a Charles Dickens tale. As an adolescent, her running was away from home and authorities. Having lost her leg hopping trains at age fourteen, she did not start running competitively until age forty. At forty-two, she set the world record for a female amputee running a marathon. Three years later, Lindsay made the Paralympic team and in Australia set records in championships for disabled athletes.

At forty-nine, a number of marathons to her credit, Lindsay wanted to do something especially "studly" [her word] for turning fifty. Despite feeling terror of water and not knowing how to swim, she decided on a triathlon. That meant overcoming aquaphobia, and beginning her very full days, training at 4:00 in the morning during a frigid Minnesota winter.

Lindsay had learned the power of breath modulation for her biking and running and began experiencing it in a significant way in her swimming. Having witnessed (with less than delight) other people breaking her records, she felt primed and pumped to create a record no one could break. To heck with a regular triathlon. *Why not become the first female amputee to complete an Ironman?* Besides the full marathon of 26.2 miles, add a 2.4-mile swim and 112-mile bike ride: grueling for any athlete, but inconceivably arduous for someone wearing a prosthesis. Lindsay would understand, almost too well, why nobody had yet achieved that record. In the meantime, she and her longtime running partner and cherished friend, Lisa, began strenuous training for the event.

On an unusually hot Ironman day, after swimming, biking, and only a few miles short of the marathon finish, Lindsay felt exhausted. Her husband Jeffrey and son Maliq were waiting for her on the sidelines. Since Lisa had passed her earlier, Lindsay asked them if she'd already crossed the line. They informed her that no, mid-marathon, Lisa had been rushed to the emergency room with kidney failure. It had appeared dire, but her husband calling from the hospital assured Jeffrey that she would live. The blazing sun and high humidity were causing competitors to collapse. She never imagined that one of them would be her partner. Reeling from the news, throbbing where her prosthesis rubbed raw, and aching throughout her entire body, Lindsay questioned whether she could continue.

Knowing his wife almost better than she knew herself, Jeffrey was sure she could; if she didn't, she'd regret it all her life. He encouraged her: "That is what Lisa would want." Her son Maliq began to run with her.

This support, incomparable willpower, and mastery of her breath propelled her forward. As she finally approached the finish line, the loudspeaker blared, beseeching the crowd to cheer in Lindsay Nielsen, *the first woman amputee in the world to complete an Ironman!* The crowd went wild. It didn't matter whether they knew her or not; tears flowed. Lindsay had another record—this one, no one could ever break.

When I asked Lindsay later what role breath played in her achievements, she responded immediately: "Breath is everything!"

Lindsay's story is a hard act to follow. Nevertheless, I will share one of my own because there are many ways to be a "good sport" other than being the best or first.

As a child, I was not athletic. My small school didn't offer sports for girls, and my speed, dexterity, and drive lacked luster. For games at recess, I was never one of the first chosen. Surprisingly, coming across a book on yoga (quite scarce then), I discovered an alternative niche.

I learned from yoga that breath coordination with movement was important. I've already related that it wasn't until I started trekking in the Himalayas and Andes that I really realized *how* important. There in the high mountains, I met my most remarkable breath teachers—they were awe-inspiring, mesmerizing, and exquisitely impressive. They also were not human. Before you start imagining that I encountered intelligent and inaccessible aliens, or perhaps dazzling, disembodied beings of light (although that would make a really good story), let me tell you I did not. My teachers were the lofty mountains themselves.

They needed no lesson plans. They were just there in all their weighty, weathered, wild, and wondrous majesty. Author of *Voices of our Ancestors,* Dhyani Ywahoo urges, "Listen to the breath and know it is the mountain's breath."

Being in their presence taught me more than any teacher or technique, how to expand lung capacity by breathing through the nose and executing full, deep yogic Complete Breaths. Sure, if I breathed through the mouth, I might be able to have some episodes of "sprinting" (as much as you can sprint in high altitude), but it wouldn't be long before I needed to stop and gasp for air. I soon learned that moving more slowly, often one breath to one step, allowed me to more fully expand the cavities of my lungs and get my breath deeper in my belly to garner more stamina. At the end of the day, it was always about stamina and not just the physical kind. Many athletes experience this. Our bodies have phenomenal abilities, but physical accomplishments often depend on whether our bodies and breath are in sync with our minds and emotions.

In 1985 I went to trek in the Himalayas of Nepal for the first time. I was a little leery but wanted to do something special and challenging to prove that in entering my thirties I wasn't over the hill yet. The altitude and the rigors of the climbs made me acutely aware of the power of breathing consciously with each step. It seemed to me to be a metaphor for life. If breath is life, then it seemed natural that consciously breathing could empower one to take the next "step" needed or desired in life.

Feeling emboldened from the new understanding of the power in my breath, the next step I desired was to feel like an athlete. If my breath had gotten me up and down those mountains, I figured it could get me through a race. Turning thirty seemed perfect timing to try a triathlon. A mini-triathlon that is: about a half-mile swim, twelve-mile bike ride, and three-mile run. Compared to an Ironman: easy peasy. Lindsay could've done it in her sleep.

Between returning from Nepal and the competition event, I had two weeks to train and learn to change gears of a borrowed speed bike. (I'd only ridden a one-speed.) I never had learned how to swim with my face in the water. Triathlon day arrived. In the midst of all the flailing arms and legs, I think my head was the only one trying to navigate above water.

Not a strong swimmer, runner, or biker, I did it for the sheer joy of participating in something I never felt I could do. I have no idea what my timing was. It didn't matter. Obviously, I wasn't the fastest and, since so many swimmers did the full triathlon, I didn't appear to be the slowest. For one morning, I felt like an athlete; enjoying the sheer exuberance of being cheered onward, and the camaraderie of hundreds of others striving for the same goal—our breath, consciously or unconsciously fueling each movement.

Scientists tell us that 70 percent of our energy comes from our breathing. For everyone, but especially for athletes, increasing oxygen levels in our bloodstream is essential to increasing the energy available in our minds and muscles. Most sports enthusiasts agree that it's both physical power and mental focus that create a true athlete. Both are enhanced by breath practice. I didn't learn this from sports, from trying to be the fastest—"the hare." I embodied it from trekking, from going leisurely but steadily—the "tortoise."

The next year, I signed up again for the mini-triathlon. The day before, I found out I could no longer use the borrowed ten-speed. Feeling at ease being "the tortoise," I decided to roll with it anyway, albeit much, *much* more slowly, with my one-speed. I was so far behind, it felt like I was ahead. It's possible I hold the distinction of the slowest record. Most important for me was the experience and the sense of athleticism. Whether last or not, I had a blast and felt like a winner.

Olympic gold medalist, Jesse Owens, asserted, "[Winning] starts with complete command of the fundamentals. Then it takes desire, determination, discipline, and self-sacrifice. And finally, it takes a great deal of love, fairness, and respect for your fellow man. Put all these together, and even if you don't win, how can you lose?"

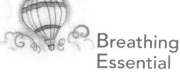

Breathing
Essential

The "whole-*BE*ing-stamina" required for high performance can be strengthened by cultivating Simple Breath Awareness throughout your everyday routines.

BLIPP

Depending on your sport or activity, practice maintaining your breath in your lower belly, or if movement and speed of motion allow, perform conscious Complete Breaths (For example, Belly Breaths for running, Complete Breaths for golf.) If possible and when comfortable, add Breath Geometry.

chapter thirty

Fear of "Flying"

Breathing for Courage

"And the trouble is, if you don't risk anything, you risk even more."
● Erica Jong, *Fear of Flying* ●

Flying, dentists, heights, public speaking, intimacy, failure, success, etc.—an endless list of fears can be helped by breathing. Lisa, a Delta flight attendant, has used breath to calm passengers feeling anxious during takeoffs, turbulence, and landings, or feeling outright panic at the sudden realization that they're strapped into a metal container hurtling through clouds at 35,000 feet. After 9/11 many flight crews themselves were affected by fear of flying. Some took leaves of absence, some took tranquilizers, and some began working with their breath.

Thich Nhat Hanh, in his book, *Peace Is Every Breath: A Practice for Our Busy Lives,* used the metaphor of an airplane when he wrote about breath, "Whenever severe turbulence comes along, the seatbelt keeps you from getting thrown around the cabin. *Mindful breathing is your seatbelt in everyday life.*"

A dentist I know has made it policy to have his patients work with their breath before he enters the room. Depending upon the patient's age and the procedure, his assistant will immediately engage them in calming breathing techniques and reminders throughout the appointment. Nancy, amazing and enthusiastic cofounder of BreathLogic, listens to a breath meditation in place of Novocain, and as surgical preop preparation and postop healing.

For many people, the number-one fear, over medical procedures, even over death, is speaking in public. And I've been there—absolutely terrified, panicked, and petrified. In fact, add humiliated, horrified, and mortified. I would rather have been in a coffin six feet under or in an urn on the mantle than on that stage!

Before I describe the specific occasion, I'll fill you in on some background. Being in front of people never came easily for me. I had to force myself to speak in front of others—prepare, practice, and pray that I would not die. I desperately wanted to address audiences because I had things I felt urged to share, so little by little I faced the fear—the anxiety, trembling, and sweating that engulfed me when I merely thought about doing it.

When I started teaching, presenting workshops, and accepting short speaking engagements, I began to practice weeks ahead, interspersing breathing techniques with the information I wanted to remember and convey in order to calm myself, focus, and retain details. I practiced Alternate Nostril Breathing right up to start time, then I began whatever session I was presenting with calming breathing techniques. I did this first for myself, as a way to slow my racing heart, but I began to see that doing so created a type of magic for everyone. Mindful breathing calmed each individual and changed the collective energy, connecting everyone on a subtle but powerful level of joining minds with hearts that set a receptive stage for whatever came next.

On New Year's Eve of 2000, in a Minneapolis venue, the stage was set, and I was on it. I had organized a fundraiser for an NGO in Guatemala where my future husband (George) and I were working.

He and his boss (two people I really did not want to fail in front of) were in the audience. I would love to tell you that I extemporaneously and eloquently so electrified the audience, painting poignant pictures of the beautiful children, hardworking families, and worthy projects that the touched, tearful audience opened wide their hearts and pocketbooks.

Nope. Never happened. I'd made the miserable mistake of not knowing exactly what I was going to say about the amazing children and families. I thought words would just come. Well they didn't. I stood speechless. I could not utter, stutter, or stammer. Nothing came out. Not a word, sentence, or syllable. Some people at first wondered if I was doing this for effect—until they got bored or embarrassed for me.

Despite my predicament, though, because of countless hours of practice, I kept my breath in my belly, so at least I didn't crumble to the ground. Although mute, I stayed present enough to lock eyes with people and maintain threads of connection. I witnessed puzzlement, compassion, and also reflected discomfort—mine feeling a hundred times stronger. After what seemed like forever, my angel friend Michele rescued me. Silently, in shame, I slithered to my seat.

After that experience, I never imagined that I could ever again get up in front of people, let alone look forward to it. Now I can laugh, but it was oh-so-painful when it happened. This was one of those experiences for which I had to practice a conscious "Let It Go" Breath. It didn't happen overnight. I needed to practice for a while. It takes courage to let things go. It takes courage to re-attempt things we've failed at. It takes courage to face fears. It takes courage at times just to get up in the morning and make it through the day. With all of these, the breath and BLIPPs are implements.

For a while, an intrepid friend Kate and I had an organization called "Transformational Journeys." With her or alone, I took groups of people on trips that tested their courage. We took journeyers out of their comfort zones, factually and symbolically. I was always astonished to see how diverse journeyers garnered the courage to utilize their breath as a tool to face new challenges. Many of those challenges involved fear of heights, literally and metaphorically. I never understood completely what bravery they had exhibited until an experience of my own.

Never *ever* having experienced a fear of heights, suddenly out of the blue, on top of Temple V, the second tallest structure in Tikal, Guatemala, I found myself in the shock of full-blown acrophobia.

Earlier I'd climbed the temple with ease, nonchalantly sitting on a ledge above the jungle canopy, watching spider monkeys play an arm's length away. However, upon approaching the ladder to descend, my stomach literally leapt into my throat. Momentarily, I felt myself teeter toward the ground, seemingly miles below.

"F*&#, I'm going to die!"

Slowly I sidled into a sitting position with my back supported against the ancient rock wall, as far from the edge as possible. As vertigo began to subside, I realized that with an invisible girdle of fear constricting my torso, I'd stopped breathing. My nervous system was a wreck. I reminded myself to breathe as deeply and consciously as possible. I needed to just sit with these sensations. Actually, I recognized helplessly, that was the only thing I could do. "Breathe low in the belly," I heard myself instructing. "It's impossible for panic to take over while breathing low in the belly."

My ego wanted to go into denial; this should *NOT* be happening to me! Yet the thought of coming near the steep staircase took my breath away. *What to do?* Alternate Nostril Breathing to the rescue! Knowing this BLIPP had always helped me gain a sense of calmness, balance, and presence; I closed my eyes and commenced a simple version.

Very soon the shock started to dissipate, and as I began to breathe easier I recalled many occasions when I'd accompanied someone to walk across a swaying bridge, approach a precipice, or ascend and descend some mountain or temple steps—Chichén-Itzá, Giza, Angkor Wat . . . step by anxious step, always counseling "Breathe!" I had felt compassion for their fears but really had no idea what they were going through. Now I understood what true bravery they'd displayed, and I doubted whether I had it myself. For a few moments, I entertained images of firemen, helicopters, and superheroes flying in to save me. Or at least to drop off a porta-potty.

No such luck.

"All right, I gotta do this!" My bladder demanded it. Thinking of the Cowardly Lion in the *Wizard of Oz,* I exhorted myself, "Ca, ca, ca ccourrraaagggge!" From somewhere in my mind I heard "Feel the fear and do it anyway!" I was definitely feeling the fear, now how to do it? I crouched down onto all fours. With a slow, deliberate exhalation orchestrated to each movement, I began crawling backward to the ladder. In this prostrated position I felt so vulnerable and humbled. Other days, on this very same temple, I'd practically sprinted to the ground while facing forward. This time my back was turned from the sky and my face kissed the staircase.

By glomming on to each stair, I tentatively began breathing my way down. With white-knuckled hands, I tightly clasped the banister as each exhale directed my foot to cautiously seek the next rung. Trepidation threatening to immobilize me was kept at bay only by each conscious breath, mated to each mindful step. I continually reminded myself of what I'd encouraged others: "Let the life force in the inhalation give you the power to let go of the fear with the exhalation, and move. If you stay conscious of your breath, and present in your body, you cannot fall." Luckily the fact that no one had ever fallen helped me loosen my iron grips to ever-so-cautiously continue.

After what seemed like a lifetime, jubilantly touching earth, I felt like kissing the ground. Great relief flooded over me. Harrowing as it was, I now savored greater empathy for others facing fears and ever-expanding gratitude for our innate abilities to courageously "breathe our way" through "ups and downs" of life.

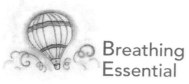

Breathing Essential

Utilizing BLIPPs proactively and in the moment (Belly Breathing, Alternate Nostril Breathing) embodies and empowers.

BLIPP

To strengthen the ability to manage panic and cultivate courage, put deposits in your breath savings account by practicing Belly Breathing often throughout your waking hours, and Alternate Nostril Breathing at least once a day.

chapter thirty-one

Breathe "Intuit"

Breathe for Intuition

Enough. These words are enough.
If not these words, this breath.
If not this breath, this sitting here.

This opening to the life
we have refused
again and again
until now.
Until now.

•   David Whyte   •

I assure you, this chapter is not "Breathe into it" misspelled. Breathing "into it" may be helpful in pain management, but "Breathe Intuit" means to feel, sense, perceive, discern, understand, and *know* at a very core level—the level to which conscious breathing can take you. The level or place of being where you are able to trust and follow your intuition as a means for decision-making, finding solutions, achieving goals, and as a leadership tool, nay—life tool!

At first reaching that level of "knowing and trusting" through breathing practice is like taking a slow walk. With practice, we learn to arrive more easily and faster, like progressing from stairs to an escalator and then elevator. When we have a question, we can breathe "intuit" and the best answer surfaces. We may feel it in our gut, know it in our heart, or sense it in our mind's eye. We are able to let go of doubt and second-guessing ourselves. We don't know how we know it's the right / best answer, or way to act, but we do. Steve Jobs advised, "Most important, have the courage to follow your heart and intuition. Somehow, they always know what you truly want to become." Intuitive Echo Bodine shares: "We need to be able to set all the voices aside, and then go to the still, small voice and say, 'show me the truth of this situation.'"

Have you ever felt the answer to some question inside you but went with another opinion, only to say, "I wish I'd followed my intuition?" The growing ability to tune into our own guidance / discernment, and then act on it, is one of the wonderful benefits of simple breath awareness practice.

Starting with just knowing when we are inhaling or exhaling helps put us in touch with our intuition. It's simple but not necessarily easy, since it requires consistent awareness and practice. Engaging deep Diaphragmatic / Belly Breathing and Complete Breath Breathing are powerful foundational practices. Adding the advanced techniques of Breath Geometry will deepen your abilities to find the presence in your body to breathe "intuit" and just know—as a sensing, perception, or feeling, be it in your gut, mind, or entire body.

Adding the gentle holdings of the Rectangle and Square Breaths to our breathing repertoire will aid in cultivating the capacity to trust what we intuit. If you can imagine yourself as a diamond, it's like you receive new facets. Other breathing BLIPPs that aid in cultivating intuition are the Heart Breath, the Relaxation Breath, and Alternate Nostril Breathing.

My cherished friend, teacher, and co-facilitator, Kirsten, always advised, "CYT—Catch Your Thoughts." A tall elegant Dane, Kirsten had moved as a young adult to Australia, where she spent decades honing her intuition and using it extensively in her healing practice. I loved co-facilitating retreats and workshops with her. Although we might have a plan of action, in sync we intuitively changed on a dime. At every event, I asked her to share a specific story about utilizing her intuition. About ten years after sharing with one attendee named Mike, he wrote to me, "Her story has stuck with me for many years and it helps me hang on when the odds are bad and the mission important."

In order to understand why Kirsten's story affected him so deeply, I am delighted to share it with you.

At age fifty, never having sailed before, Kirsten took off from the Australian coast in a catamaran with a sea-loving sailor named Mark. They were to spend years sailing around the world.

After spending many months throughout the South Pacific, they took off in the middle of the Indian Ocean from the tiny, isolated, "speck on the map" called Christmas Island. They had been cruising all day, propelled by a speedy tailwind. Now it was the wee hours, foggy, with no stars or moonlight. Kirsten was below deck, waiting for her turn "at watch" when she heard a thud, and her name called from a distance like she'd never heard it before—a bloodcurdling "Kirrrrssstteennnnnnnn!"

She dashed up and shouted, "Mark, where are you?" As the boat kept speeding onward, from the inky depths came the already distant reply, "In the waterrrrrr." Immediately the gravity of the situation took hold. Kirsten was hundreds of miles away from land, alone on a boat she did not know how to sail, her skilled companion left behind in open ocean without a buoy or life jacket.

She'd watched Mark and had helped with the sails, but for numerous reasons he'd never gotten around to teaching her how to maneuver the boat by herself. Beside herself with panic and anger that he hadn't worn a harness, she swore at him (forgive the pun) like a sailor: "You #$@&%*! How could you do this to me!"

The probabilities that she could never navigate back to

Christmas Island and that both she and Mark would perish at sea in untimely and dreadful deaths literally took her breath away. After letting her fury spill out, she realized she had to get hold of herself, calm her breath and thoughts, and decide what to do next. She recounted later that as the boat was racing away from him "terrifyingly fast," it occurred to her that she could never live with herself if she left Mark to die.

How the f*&# do I find him? she first asked herself. Then with a deep breath, Kirsten set the intention to only focus her thoughts on the most important questions:

1. Where is he?
2. How do I find him?
3. What do I do next?

Immediately her intuition had her read the compass and begin to take down the sails. With no wind power she needed to rely on the boat's motor; however it didn't work well. Whenever Mark started the motor, he had to use a big screwdriver and withstand several shocks before it clicked on.

Casting aside persistent doubt that she could do it, Kirsten stayed with her three questions, which led her down below to stimulate the second battery that started the power. Back at the helm, she was dismayed knowing she had no idea how far the boat had traveled from him. To complicate matters, in her mind the compass was 300 degrees, so in turning around, she compensated 150 degrees. Kirsten continued that trajectory for quite a while until she responded to a nagging voice in her head that continually beseeched her to "check the compass." Finally acquiescing, she grasped that it was 360 degrees and she was supposed to turn 180, not 150 degrees, and now she needed to overcompensate. How to do this?

An intuitive healer who had learned to trust her inner guidance, she asked, "Okay, whoever or whatever guides my hands and breath during treatments, guide me now!" Then Kirsten trusted implicitly that this higher direction would stop her hand on the throttle when it was right.

Steering the boat through the darkness, she lost all concept of time. Since he'd fallen, she knew it had been hours, but how many, she couldn't even guess. Suddenly her hand halted. The boat stopped. Switching on all the lights, she hollered Mark's name at the top of her lungs. After about a minute, from the distant blackness, wafted a reply. She slowly powered the boat toward his relieved and excited sounds until he swam about 25 meters to climb onboard.

Once Mark was on deck, saved from a watery death, then the calmness Kirsten had cultivated during her rescue effort disappeared completely, and she let Mark have it in no uncertain terms. She related that later, while lying in her berth, her entire body shook uncontrollably until the trauma released.

I was fortunate to hear this story also from Mark. Having gone out to fix some ropes, he'd slipped and fallen. For several seconds he desperately attempted to hold on to the edge, but arthritis in his hands forced him to let go. That's when he screamed Kirsten's name. Witnessing the boat speed away, he thought to himself, *Damn, I should've worn a harness!*

Well, I've had a good life. Now, how am I going to die? The thought occurred that even though he hadn't taught her how to sail, if there was anyone in the world who could find him, it was Kirsten. However Mark realized the odds were fully against him. He checked for open wounds that would draw sharks and finding none, settled into a back float and eventually fell asleep to conserve energy.

Having no idea how much time had passed, in what seemed like a dream, Mark thought he heard his name, though the water in his ears muffled the sound. *It's just wishful thinking,* he chided himself; but hearing it again, he opened his eyes, lifted his head, and saw in the distance: Lights!

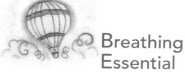

Breathing
Essential

Focusing attention on the physical movement of the breath clears and calms the mind, allowing one to connect more deeply with their intuition.

BLIPP

Practice: With a question in mind, explore various BLIPP breathing techniques, then become quiet and notice where or how you intuit your answer.

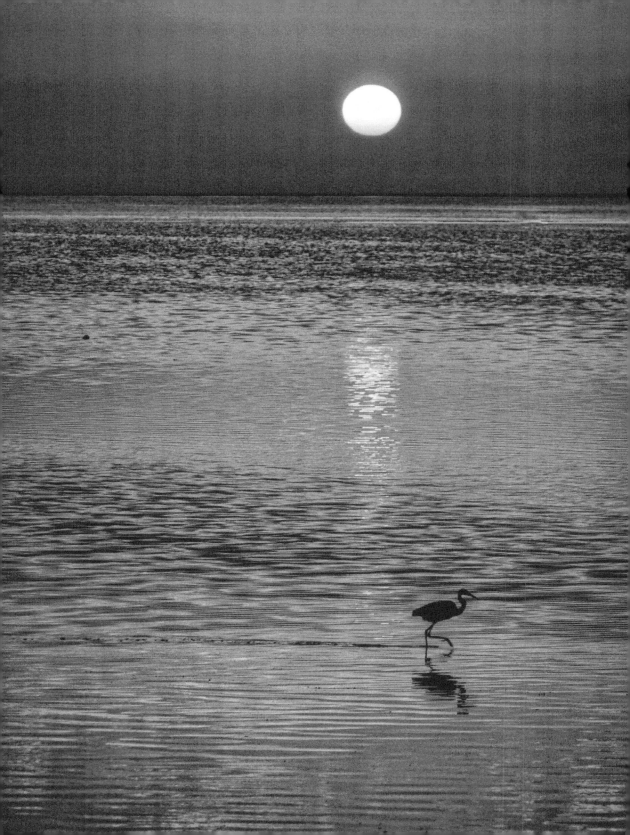

VI

breathing throughout life

chapter thirty-two

Oh, to Be Young Again!

Not All That It Seems

Stress has reached epidemic proportions in children and adolescents. According to the American Psychological Association and the American College Health Association, half of college-level students report overwhelming anxiety. Children cannot learn well when stressed; their brains shut down and information does not move from short-term to long-term memory. Studies convey that anxiety disorders begin affecting many children in elementary school and escalate in high school, often topping stress levels for adults.

Reasons and symptoms cited:

- increase in homework for young children,
- pressures of test-taking and exams,
- less time spent playing and being physically active,
- less focus on art and music,
- unstructured play time replaced with regulated activities,
- hyper-connectivity/cyber-bullying,
- unprecedented access to disturbing news, violence, sexuality, harsh realities,

- moodiness, depression, reluctance to go to school, thoughts of suicide,
- sleep deprivation,
- chronic illnesses (asthma, diabetes, obesity),
- medications once reserved for adults,
- behavioral and learning problems, and
- excessive focus on the future instead of the present.

The greatest travesty: The loss of the ease and joy of childhood. Society seems to be coercing children onto a treadmill that leads to loss of innocence, panic disorders, depression, a host of maladies, workaholism, and other addictions. *What to do?*

Certain experts recommend adding unstructured family time (preferably in nature), time spent journaling, better nutrition, earlier bedtime, less screen time, less homework, and limited social media. (Some parents can comply while many consider it impossible.) Other experts advise psychotropic drugs, psychiatrists, and psychotherapy.

BreathLogic suggests it would be helpful to integrate Breath Literacy into school curricula worldwide. A child's most important activity, bar none, is breathing! Some children are computer literate by age four but have no idea how to breathe well. Yet it's oxygen that powers their brains and feeds every cell of their developing bodies. It's time for Breath Literacy to provide a powerful foundation for all other literacies taught in schools for these reasons:

1. Breath is life, powering every activity.
2. Our breath's oxygen fuels the brain.
3. We cannot learn or perform optimally if our nervous system is not functioning well.
4. We can change our nervous system and our brain by changing our breath.
5. Practices of Breath Literacy will help aid children's:
   - overall health, stress resiliency, and sleep,
   - grounding, relaxation, moods, and energy levels,

- self-confidence, self-empowerment, empathy, and compassion, and
- focus, memory, intuition, and creativity.

My sister Susan, a retired educator who has been both an elementary teacher and principal, nationally and internationally, is a proponent of Breath Literacy. To help manage her own stress levels while elementary principal at the American Embassy School in New Delhi, she regularly worked with a breath instructor in her office after the school day. Susan kept a "breathing ball" by her desk and when children would come and visit, they breathed together. Dr. George, in his office as school psychologist, kept a "breathing ball" as a device to connect with students and help shift their nervous systems into parasympathetic dominance.

In the highly competitive schools where Susan worked she was very aware of the high stress levels for administrators, teachers, and students. Many parents fostered lofty expectations for their children's higher education upon their entering elementary school. They desired teachers to give homework that would provide the "edge" for their sons and daughters acceptance into elite universities. Being an administrator who strongly supported both the immediate and long-term needs of the "whole child," she asked for a committee to research evidence-based studies on the effects of homework for grade levels 1–5. Their findings resulted in recommendations of after-school play time, pursuits of passion, and parents deciding how families could spend their evenings in lieu of homework assignments.

The studies showed that excessive homework and the push to handle a workload out of sync with their development level led to significant stress for students and their parents. Stephanie Donaldson-Pressman, a contributing editor of a study published in *The American Journal of Family Therapy*, reports that excessive homework "is not only not beneficial to children's grades or GPA, but shows a plethora of evidence that it's detrimental to their attitudes about school, grades, self-confidence, social skills, and quality of life."

The proposal that Breath Literacy be implemented into curricula is a way to help provide the "edge" that parents desire for their children, whether privileged or not, in all schools, private or public.

Author, educator, and Breath Literacy supporter, Dr. Verna Price, is a force. Raised in the Bahamas, witnessing the struggles of her mother earning low wages as a maid fostered the desire to improve circumstances for herself and others. Education was the way.

Dr. Verna calls herself "Dr." not because she cares that others know she has a doctorate. She does care that young women of color have role models for higher education. Thus she founded Girls Taking Action (GTA); developing a curriculum to engage these students in academics and leadership, to learn how to use their personal power, think critically, develop careers, become leaders, and give back to their communities. Dr. Verna's book, *The Power of People: Four Kinds of People Who Can Change Your Life*, is required reading. From it, the girls learn to discern who acts as an "adder, subtractor, multiplier, or divider" in their lives. Her program has expanded to other schools, cities, and countries with tremendous success.

At one point, Dr. Verna decided she wanted the girls to also learn Breath Literacy, recognizing the need for their women mentors to learn it first themselves.

The girls voluntarily joining the program did not enjoy the same privileges of many other students. Often and for various reasons, their home circumstances and environments were less than stable or advantageous. These girls could uniquely benefit from utilizing the power of breath to find a peaceful sanctuary within.

As part of the GTA curriculum, mentors routinely start and end sessions with everyone enthusiastically reciting the mantra: *"I am valuable! I am important! I am lovable! I am powerful!"* Many adolescents expect value, importance, lovability, and power to come from outside themselves. Dr. Verna desired these qualities to arise from within the girls. Adding work with the breath was an empowering, effective way to do so.

"I AM valuable!" Every conscious inhale and exhale we perform "unearths the priceless, buried treasures" available in our breath.

"I AM important!" By practicing BLIPPs, we send ourselves the clear message: "Yes! I am important enough to give myself this valuable time and attention."

"I AM lovable!" Spending time focusing on our breath is a profound act of self-love and self-care; a way of developing a loving relationship with ourselves that is foundational for healthy relationships with others.

"I AM powerful!" Conscious breathing teaches us how to move from rashly reacting (our reptilian brain) to consciously responding (our developed brain). Reactivity becomes response-ability—ability to respond with deliberate choice. With responsibility comes true power, not bequeathed from the outside—but from within. Breath Literacy fosters confidence, executive functions, and leadership skills.

> "The hope of a nation lies in the proper education of its youth."
> • Erasmus •

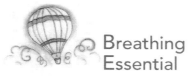

Breathing Essential

The sooner children can learn that their own breath holds powerful tools, the easier, more empowered, and stress-resilient their childhoods can be.

BLIPP

Parents and teachers can model "pausitivity" and breath awareness by periodically asking their children or students to stop for a moment to:

- Notice a full cycle of breath (or several cycles).
- Breathe out any stress, and breathe in peace.
- Perform a long sigh, then notice a deeper inhale.

chapter thirty-three

Breath Literacy and BBH

The Brain, Breath, and Heart

Dr. George adds:

There has been much research over the last twenty-five years on a special class of neurons found in a number of areas of the brain: frontal lobe and several areas of the parietal lobe. Called "mirror neurons," they were discovered serendipitously while Italian researchers were studying macaque monkeys. The researchers found that these specific neurons activated in two different ways:

1. They fired when a behavior was executed.
2. They fired also when a behavior was only observed.

Growing research suggests that humans experience similar responses. An article in *Neuroscience News*, April 2019, reported, "Human neuroimaging studies have shown that when we experience pain ourselves, we activate a region of the brain called the cingulate cortex. When we see someone else in pain, we activate the same region." These mirror neurons may be a neurological explanation for how we can "walk in another person's shoes." This has huge implications for understanding how children and adults may "read" the emotional states of others and experience empathy—the ability to share and understand another's feelings.

Through the process and function of both neuroception and mirror neurons, we have the ability to intentionally and consciously manage our nervous system and the nervous systems of others. Numerous times when I was a school psychologist, adolescents ran into my room panicked because something "terrible" had happened. Their breathing was fast and shallow, their faces expressing fear, anger, or confusion, as they struggled to manage their internal experience and seek support.

By intentionally using my voice (gentle and prosodic), soft eye contact, compassionate facial expression, gestures, and spatial boundaries that suggested safety, my nervous system was able to calm them. This approach, along with gentle but firm suggestions to breathe slowly and into their belly, was an opportunity to teach self-soothing.

After a few sessions of this gentle attunement, many students were able to internalize my voice, support, and care, and begin to provide this for themselves—to self-regulate and shift from sympathetic to parasympathetic activation. I believe this occurred because they felt safe and also unconsciously reflected or mimicked (mirror neurons) what they were experiencing in my nervous system.

These dynamics happen elsewhere as well. I was called into a classroom where previously calm and attentive students were suddenly "acting out." The teacher had no explanation since their parents indicated there were no problems at home. I observed this classroom several times and noticed a number of students struggling with age-appropriate self-control and executive functions. After closer observation, I began to perceive anxiety and frustration on the part of the teacher. Normally quite serene, caring, and emotionally present with her students, she now appeared impatient and emotionally absent. In private she shared that she was in the middle of a very painful divorce, with her inner world "deeply shaken." I wondered out loud if her students, like a barometer, might be absorbing some of her anxiety and discomfort. Was it possible that her students were feeling unsafe emotionally and reflecting some of her anxiety, confusion, anger, and sadness?

Upon tracing back when her students started to "act out," she realized they were mirroring her own feelings. Once she appreciated how important she was personally to the stability of her classroom, along with the impact of her emotional state, with some support she began managing her own nervous system, thereby positively affecting the classroom dynamics.

It is an extremely powerful experience to become aware of the impact of our psychological and emotional states.

Aristotle declared, "Educating the mind without educating the heart is no education at all." BreathLogic adds, "Educating the mind and the heart without educating about the breath misses the golden link. Educating the mind and heart along with the breath connects the golden link."

DEEPENING TIP: The heart and brain communicate with each other through the neck. Take time throughout the day to relieve tension in the area of your neck and shoulders. Examples: slow conscious neck rolls, massage, shaking practice.

Do you remember the tale about the Brain, Breath, and Heart in chapter 1? Well this time, they go into the school cafeteria to discuss which one is most important for a child's educational success.

The Brain orders a double espresso and booms, "I am the brain! Without me children cannot develop their minds, nor advance academically. There's no contest. I AM THE MOST IMPORTANT!"

The Heart sips tomato juice and softly responds, "Yes, dear, wonderful Brain, you are essential for knowledge; but with all due respect, if children in a classroom are feeling lonely, rejected, unsafe, or bullied, they are not happy, and happy children learn better. In settings where social-emotional learning (SEL), which I direct, is emphasized, studies relate results of greater academic achievement, *kindness and love.*" The Heart humbly affirms, "I am the most important!"

The Breath stops drinking from a large glass of oxygen-rich water and sighs a deep, breathy, slow sigh. (Remember how the Breath loves to sigh?) "*Ahhhhhhhhhhhhh,* Dear Brain and Dear Heart, you are each amazing and essential to a child's educational success! I can't imagine a classroom without you both! I remind you though, I am the fuel that powers your functions. Practicing Breath Literacy enhances my abilities to augment *your* abilities, thus attaining ideal educational success! In fact, let's drop this competition and instead collaborate together in considering the whole child. Not just his or her academic or social-emotional success, but life success. I propose that you utilize me as the golden link to create a powerful synergy, greater than any of us alone.

"Let's co-create innovative curricula that integrates the expertise of Breath Literacy with evidence-based benefits of mindfulness, physical movement, SEL, peace studies, and the latest in neuropsychology for children. By joining together, we can provide educators and students with the grade-specific programs that can enhance and realize each child's highest potential for learning and well-being. We shall call it the Brain, the Breath, and the Heart (BBH), and more than a whole-child approach, it will be a whole-school approach. Improving student well-being necessitates improving well-being for teachers, administrators, parents, and the school. BBH will bring forth a whole systems change."

Teachers and administrators live in "overwhelm," with thirty billion things they fit into a mere day. If you've ever known an educator, you've witnessed the toxic toll of walloping workloads and endless expectations. There are times of the year they are just running on empty. And, that's just it! *Run on empty no more!* Breath is our fuel, sustenance, and power! The Brain, the Breath, and the Heart (BBH) is a "lifeline," not only for breath awareness but for breathing optimally to utilize our body's and brain's most valuable sustenance: oxygen.

FACT REMINDER: Our brains weigh only about 2 percent of our total body weight, yet utilize about 20 percent or more of our body's total circulating oxygen.

The key is to incorporate "refueling" in simple and consistent BLIPPs throughout the day as part of education protocol. The last thing an educator needs is another item on their to-do list. Educators need to understand not how to DO a lifeline—but how to BE a lifeline for themselves, and then disseminate this "way of BEing" to their pupils and the student body as a whole.

Therefore, we propose a "To-Be" list which includes:

- *Be* more calm, peaceful, and balanced.
- *Be* more focused to better concentrate, assimilate, and retain information.
- *Be* more kind, compassionate, and open-hearted.
- *Be* more alert, energized, and revitalized.
- *Be* more self-assured, confident, and empowered.

"If we want to change the world, we must begin with the children."
• Gandhi •

Students' well-being is directly linked to their teachers' well-being. The more grounded and balanced the educator, the more grounded and balanced the student, leading to an optimal learning environment. BBH provides educators with a foundational practice in breathing techniques that can easily become a healthy, empowering way of being and functioning—first for themselves, then for students, parents, and families. And we are not being highfalutin by believing the results will reverberate around the world. These techniques (many BLIPPs) can be inserted into established curricula in ten-second to ten-minute blocks of time throughout the day, helping to revitalize educators and students.

Introduction of such a practice can be done at the beginning of the school year, in one session, or preferably a number of days or weeks.

The teacher initiates an art project with the students exploring the word "BREATHE." First they discuss what the word means: why breathing is important (the science, physiology, and cross-curriculum applications, depending on grade level and personal experiences). They spend selected time frames working with each letter, learning specific BLIPP techniques for what each letter stands for, and how and when they can utilize them to enhance scholastic and life experiences. After discussion of each letter, the students integrate the dynamics of what they've learned by crafting or designing each letter.

Belly Relax Energize Attention Trees Heart Empower

At the end of the lessons the finished art project reminds them of different reasons and ways to *breathe* to enhance their learning and lives. This provides a powerful platform for integrating BLIPPs into curricula and daily routines, while also spontaneously utilizing them in specific situations for calming, energizing, or focusing. Adding Breath Literacy to curricula will have a profound, positive impact.

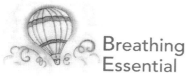

Breathing Essential

Oxygen powers the brain and aids all learning and executive functions.

BLIPP

Practice "B R E A T H E." For a selected time period, focus on BLIPP practices for one letter at a time.

chapter thirty-four

Recapping with the Three N's

Nurture, Nourish, Nature

"From Wakan Tanka, the Great Spirit,
there came a great unifying life force
that flowed through all things—
the flowers of the plants,
blowing winds,
rocks, trees, birds, animals—
and it was the same force
that had been breathed into the first man."
• Oglala Sioux •

As we are nearing the end of our Breath Literacy course, it's a good time to recap and also explore a few more nuances of how "breath is life."

NURTURE

Throughout this book, Dr. George has explained how our nervous system and breath intricately relate to aspects of safety. In psychologist Abraham Maslow's hierarchy of needs, physiological necessities and then safety form the base of his pyramid. Safety and the experience of being nurtured are foundational for well-being as a platform for growth throughout life. Think of a fetus being incubated in a womb and then swaddled and nurtured upon birth. For the newborn, safety and nurturance are synonymous with mama. We never grow out of this need. As we age, we usually search to meet these needs in many ways and by many people. Ideally we learn to get these needs met notably within ourselves.

By being present with our breath, we can nurture ourselves on the supportive level of a parent, friend, partner, lover, counselor, or therapist. We can accompany and witness ourselves on a deep, energetic level. As Dr. George has shown in psychological parlance, we learn to self-soothe, an invaluable practice that will serve us throughout life. Not just when someone "takes our toy," but when people don't act the way we want them to, our plans don't turn out the way we expect, and all kinds of shit and shift happen. We might not be able to control circumstances, but we can, with our breath, control the way we respond and how circumstances affect us. Jonathan Lockwood Huies, "Philosopher of Happiness," wrote, "Perhaps today is a day to soothe your ruffled feathers, take a deep breath, and reaffirm that the weight of the world is really not on your shoulders . . ."

For a moment, even as you read, bring your attention to the physical movement of your breath. Feel when you are inhaling, and feel when you are exhaling. Notice the profound sense of constant care that your breathing ceaselessly provides. Can you sense your breath as a consistent, nurturing companion on your life's journey?

Ahhhhhhhhhhhhhhhhhhhh, your breath is no imaginary friend; it is real, tangible, healing, and something you never outgrow. You can make breath a best friend that is always there for you. The more you nurture your breath, the greater care it will take of you and provide you a safe refuge throughout your life.

NOURISH

Imagine for a moment that you are in the womb that bore you. We know that fetuses receive the sustenance they need from their mothers through the umbilical cord. In the West, this is seen as purely nutritional. In the East, it is seen as nutritional and also energetic—both equal in importance.

After we are born, we receive most nutrition from our food, but also energetic nutrients from the elements of earth, air, fire (sun) and water, our breath acting as an umbilical cord or conduit through which our bodies receive them. How we nourish ourselves by both food and prana (life force) of the breath is essential to creating optimal well-being. Vitamins, minerals, and nutrients from food are fuel that nourishes us on a physical level. Our breath/prana is fuel nourishing us on more subtle, energetic, and spiritual levels—life as a miracle, mystery, gift, opportunity, adventure, and conscious creation.

Physician, psychotherapist, and developer of bioenergetic analysis, Alexander Lowen asserted, "We live in an ocean of air, like fish in a body of water. By our breathing, we are attuned to our atmosphere. If we inhibit our breathing, we isolate ourselves from the medium in which we exist. In all oriental and mystic philosophies, the breath holds the secret to the highest bliss."

Author Dennis Lewis adds, "When we are able to breathe through our whole body, sensing our verticality from head to foot, we are aligning ourselves with the natural flow of energy connecting heaven and earth."

NATURE

"And into the forest I go, to lose my mind and find my soul."
•   John Muir   •

Where you live, you might not have access to a forest, but find nature in any way, shape, or form. Even if it's buying some "Lucky Bamboo" that doesn't need much light to grow. Surround yourself as much as possible with living, breathing and growing plants and greenery. Studies report that blood pressure drops, cortisol levels decrease, and moods elevate. It is an unequivocal fact that we need nature for our well-being.

Simply and powerfully, trees are the lungs of our planet. Spending time amidst trees has known scientific benefits. The Japanese call it "forest bathing." Unfortunately, humans have been cutting down trees and Rainforests at the rate of six football fields a minute, a country the size of Panama every year. We cannot offer a book on breath without addressing this issue. Humans are essentially destroying the life force of the planet, with direct repercussions for our breath and our lives. I'd like to share an experience that made these statistics personal.

Before the millennium, at a conference in Wisconsin, I translated for two Guarani shamans from Paraguay. They met with Native American leaders to discuss our planetary situation going forward into the next century and what it meant for indigenous peoples and our Earth. The meetings were joyous, painful, dire, uplifting, inspirational, depressing, and hopeful—all at once. After that week, I was invited to visit the shamans in their communities.

In Paraguay a month later, Ramon, the shaman's translator between Guarani and Spanish, my close friend Jan, and I began a cross-country bus ride, from Asuncion, in the west, to near the Brazilian border in the east.

Imagine please that you are on that bus with us. We begin our odyssey before dawn with the windows open, listening to a concert of myriad birds and countless species of animals. The awakening jungle vibrates with sounds of chirrups, chirping, squawks, caws, chattering, croaks, howls, buzzing, tweeting, trills, hissing, and hums wafting all around us. Shadows of wild and lush beauty become delineated with the rising sun. We watch families of monkeys swinging across branches with ease and daring.

Attention shifts between exquisite scenery outside and companions inside. Not far down the road with a lull in conversation, we abruptly become aware of an eerie quiet outside. The ubiquitous animal sounds are gone! Fertile smells of sumptuous vegetation are missing, and our bewildered eyes suddenly behold land that looks like the Midwestern plains! The line of demarcation separating the jungle and the clear-cutting stretches before us. The cool shade of the canopy of thousands of trees is replaced by blazing sun.

For the majority of the trip, for hours upon hours, for as far as the eye can see, we rumble across land that was once verdant Rainforest, a haven to thousands of species of animals, trees, foliage, and insects. That vibrant existence now extinguished. The only life we see are grazing cattle as silence assaults our ears. We feel collective pain.

That ride affected me deeply. My heart ached seeing the destruction I'd known existed but only in glimpses. My mind knew the statistics—numbers I really couldn't wrap my head around, but now my heart understood. Millions of trees had been cut down in what felt like massacre for the forests, and slow suicide for humans, the "magic" in our air disappearing.

I knew what we had witnessed was only a small example of the Rainforests and wildlife vanishing all over the planet at an alarming rate. During twelve consecutive years of trekking in Nepal, and thirty years of travel or living in Guatemala, I continually observed effects of widespread deforestation.

With all my heart, I feel we can and must change this trajectory.

Trees=Breath
Breath=Us
Earth–Trees=No Us

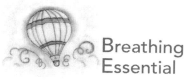

Breathing Essential

Trees are as important to us as life itself.

BLIPP

Wherever you are, as often as possible, surround yourself with nature and trees (even if only in your imagination). Consciouly breathe as you:

- Hug a tree.
- Gaze at a tree.
- Climb a tree.
- Sit in a tree.
- Draw a tree.
- Plant a tree.

chapter thirty-five

The Golden Years

Breathing as We Age

Have you heard about the seeker who spent a life savings to travel and find an ancient sage high in a Himalayan cave? After many trials and tribulations, when finally found, the wise man informed the seeker there could be one question only. Without hesitation, the intrepid inquirer implored, "Oh great master, please tell me the secret to a long life?"

With a sigh, the two-word response came immediately: "Keep breathing."

This may seem anticlimactic, but it's true. An African proverb goes, "Life is your ability to breathe out every time you breathe in." According to philosopher Gurdjieff, "Time is breath." As long as you're breathing, you're alive. One of the great benefits of learning Breath Literacy when younger is that as one grows older in age, life force is still vibrant in the body. Quality of breath helps determine quality of life, especially as we age. For many, what is supposed to be the "golden" years can feel more like "rusty tin." But hopefully, with the utilized life force of the breath, as Betty Friedan theorized, "Aging is not lost youth but a new stage of opportunity and strength."

If there is openness and desire, it is never too late to develop and benefit from Breath Literacy. Elders are a population so dear to my heart, and I am certain that practicing Breath Literacy will add quality to the quantity of their years.

As a child I remember hearing my dad conjecture to my mom (along with the Beatles), whether she'd still need him and still feed him *"when I'm sixty-four?"* That age, seeming ancient then, now feels like the prime of life. My six years younger mother, took loving care of him until he was ninety. The last two years of his life, he barely breathed. He'd fallen, broken his hip, and had a colostomy. Dad never voiced a word of complaint, but we knew he was depressed; his breathing imperceptible. He had been diagnosed with a rare leukemia but died from a burst bowel. I witnessed his agony when it happened. The ambulance couldn't come quickly enough.

For many elders and people who, for various reasons, are scarcely breathing, stagnant air in the lungs becomes toxic to their bodies and results in slow poisoning. This is what happened to my father. When most people ponder the importance of their breath—very seldom do they think about the functions of ventilation and massage produced by the physical movement of the breath. (Functions aided greatly by Diaphragmatic/Belly Breaths, Complete Breaths, and Breath Geometry.)

Imagine going into a closed room that has been "hermetically sealed" for many years. Does the stagnant air affronting you make you want to hold your breath or gag? Imagine now being stuck between floors, hours and even days, in a small elevator (like those in old hotels that can barely fit one person with luggage). Yes you'd be hungry (hopefully you packed some snacks), but more importantly, very soon, with the lack of ventilation you would be recycling only foul air. Even if you did have enough food and water to remain a week, month, or year, your vital organs and body systems would begin closing down because of the torpid toxicity of the less-than-fresh air.

This scenario is analogous to the experience of sedentary elders and others who are incapacitated, bedridden, or in wheelchairs. Although the accommodations are hopefully better than an elevator, their breath does not ventilate the lungs, so the same sorry semblance of air stagnates in their lungs for months and even years. The breath's tasks of purifying the blood with fresh oxygen and eliminating carbon dioxide can barely be performed. Putrid air devoid of life force seeps into our vital organs, acting as a slow poisoning. Roman author, Ovid, stressed, "Sickness seizes the body from bad ventilation."

Have you ever had a massage? If so, you know it can be pure heaven. If you've never had one, now's the time, and don't be afraid to ask for it to be more gentle or strong. Afterward while you are invigorated, yet melting from relaxation and sensual pleasure, you will understand how your organs feel from your breath's inner massage.

Champion athlete Paul Bragg told us: "Shallow breathers poison themselves." Inner massage is one of the major tasks our respiration needs to perform. The diaphragm, intercostal muscles, and subsidiary muscles in the torso that are utilized during deep breathing, massage and knead our vital organs and glands, aiding them to function better and maintain homeostasis. These movements release tension and enhance the performance of all body systems. The best inside ventilation and massage is deep belly laughter and Complete Breath Breathing. The best outside ventilation and massage are nature's breezes and loving hands.

One of the reasons I am so passionate about sharing better breathing practices with elders is because of experiences with my parents as they aged.

I mentioned that my mother was a nurse. As a child, I visited the nursing home where she worked and heard residents call her their "angel in white." Mom loved "the old people," and they loved her.

When training new staff, she always urged them to treat the residents with utmost respect and give them the care they would want their parents, grandparents, or someday themselves to receive.

Although she meted out plenty of pills, she herself refused medication until after age eighty. Always wary of side effects, she acquiesced only after a diagnosis of high blood pressure. During one visit home, I watched her worriedly take her blood pressure several times in one hour. I observed her shallow, rapid, upper chest breathing and understood how it escalated her hypertension and contributed to her panic. For years I'd wanted to work with her, but she'd always declared, "I know how to breathe! I've been doing it all my life!"

She could not fathom that breath should be given special attention. There was never any reference to proper breathing in her medical training.

It occurred to me that showing her something tangible might make a difference. I asked her to check my blood pressure. She fitted me with the cuff, turned on the device and upon receiving the numbers exclaimed: "Oh, Laurie, what excellent blood pressure you have!"

"Thank you, Mom!" I graciously smiled and said, "I want you to see what happens to my blood pressure when I breathe like you've been breathing." For ninety seconds, I breathed only in my upper chest, shallowly and erratically. It felt awful to me, but was worth it. My blood pressure shot up, and Mom saw it.

Then I continued, "Now, look what happens when I do low, slow belly breathing." After another ninety seconds, my mother saw with her own eyes how my blood pressure came down.

"Well, I'll be!" she exclaimed. "Can you show me how to do that?"

Immediately, before she could change her mind, we started working. And we worked. And we worked. It took time for her to gain new breathing habits, but I am so grateful she was determined. As a result, Mom understood that if she began to feel anxious for any reason she needed to immediately get her breath in her belly. In her nineties, she made sure her caregivers knew how to instruct her in case she went into panic mode and forgot. She became convinced that breathing better added both quality and quantity time to the end of her life.

I want everyone's grandparents, parents, and all of us, as we journey through the years, to enjoy the highest quality of life possible. Can you imagine the impact Breath Literacy could have in assisted living, nursing homes, or home-care environments?

First, all staff would be trained in Breath Literacy for their own self-care and to manage compassion fatigue. Being proactive in preventing professional burnout is essential in promoting patient care. Staff cannot provide quality care when feeling depleted. As with educators, busy caregivers do not need another thing "To Do." The key: integrate Breath Literacy as a way "To BE" personally and professionally.

Second, staff would be trained in how to share Breath Literacy and BLIPPs with their residents. Ideally, special personnel will implement supportive, sustainable programming to realize the greatest positive impact for all concerned.

Statistics relay that lung capacity begins to decline after about age thirty-five. The diaphragm loses power, intercostal muscles and tissues lose elasticity, alveoli weaken, rib-cage bones change shape, the brain's messages to the lungs are not as strong. What does this all mean? *Unless we are actively exercising our muscles of respiration, we are decreasing the amount of oxygen moving in and carbon dioxide moving out of the bloodstream.* Quality of breath deteriorates, and we know where that leads: the slippery slope of shallow breathing!

It may seem like we're headed for doom, destruction, and demise, but take a breath, savor, and sigh, for all is not lost! Remember that breathing savings account we advised you to start in chapter 6? The golden years are the time to cash in. And most importantly to continue "saving." Statistics report that people are living longer and longer.

"Financial" planning advice for graceful aging: Keep putting "deposits" into your "pension." Remember what Sophia Loren advised: "Posture!" Also walk! Sing! Move your arms! Loosen / shake! Dance! As the wise sage says, "Keep breathing." Let's keep breathing better—not just for surviving but for thriving!

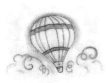

Breathing
Essential

Breath is life. The quality of our lives as we age is directly impacted by the quality of our breath. Just watching our breath deepens our breath.

BLIPP

Daily, choose specific ways and times to watch your breath.

chapter thirty-six

'Till Death Do Us Part

Breathing for the End of Life

Have you heard the maxim: "If you haven't experienced death, you haven't really experienced life"? Whether true or not, death is a part of life, and the way one breathes with those who are dying is extremely important. Final breaths are a very significant stage of life, and an important juncture for those accompanying them. Some people die rapidly and others die gradually with lingering last breaths. These ultimate breaths, however few or many they may be, as a clinging to life, or a letting go of life, can be precious for all involved.

Let's talk about dying. A deep bow of gratitude to Dr. Elizabeth Kubler-Ross for her pioneering work to make dying respectable, and to help loved ones better understand grief. Sometime in the 1960s, the nursing home where my mother worked sent her to a conference on death and dying put on by Dr. Kubler-Ross. My mother had never been to a conference. She came back energized and transformed with renewed commitment to caregiving and spending quality time with each resident. She saw her role in a new way, as a type of midwife supporting and easing the dying from one existence to another, whatever that existence may be.

Dying persons in hospitals used to be hidden, and the death of a patient was considered a failure instead of a natural progression. John B. Goodman in his book, *The Road to Self*, talks about death as a transition, something to look forward to. As an owner of assisted-living homes for elders, he was a pioneer in desiring to bring breath practices to staff and residents. Individuals who specialize in hospice care, and those who are enlisted because of relationship, soon learn the importance of being present and consciously breathing with their patients and loved ones.

Ideally patients have engaged in breath practices while alive and healthy. That may not be the case though, nor would it be the time to give "how to" lessons. If people in the room are scared or anxious, you don't even have to say a word. As Dr. George has shown how one nervous system can manage others, one's manner of breathing can help create a more conscious, calm ambiance. Caroline Goydor in her TEDx talk asks, "How do you know who the most powerful person in the room is? An actor will tell you it's about the breath. The most powerful person in the room has the most relaxed breathing pattern."

How you breathe when you are with someone who is preparing to leave this world is very significant and also very simple. It is all about your quality of presence; leaving your agenda, to-do lists, and any outside concerns behind. Focus fully on being in the present moment from a place of groundedness, heartfulness, and peacefulness. Let your breath be deep, slow, and conscious. You can imagine breathing in and out through your heart. Barbara McAfee, author of *Full Voice, The Art and Practice of Vocal Presence*, has shared poignantly, how the breathing done while singing helped to ease her mother's transition experience.

Dr. George adds:

As long as we live, we can make every breath count.

Changes in our brains occur when we are alert, focused, and motivated; the ideal requirements of learning and living, no matter what age. This combination of attention and intention makes good music and through repetition (the practice of new thoughts, attitudes, and actions) will lead to building new neural networks or highways in the brain. Whether we are a child, teen, adult, or elder, this allows us to continue to create "new musical scores" instead of constantly playing the same negative, depressed, or scary song in our head, day in and day out. In this way we can consciously utilize our prefrontal cortex and executive functions to provide us more options and freedom to be who we wish to be in our relationships and life experiences until our dying day.

The practices and strategies described in this book are very potent; together they can have a transformative impact on all aspects of our lives to the final breath.

When my dear friend Juanita, a nurse, advocate of breath practices, and a devoted supporter and board member for BreathLogic, was dying, I asked her constantly what I could do for her. Her consistent answer was, "Breathe with me."

Breathe with Me

Give me the gift
of your presence
Breathe with me

Nothing more to say
Nothing more to do
Just breathe with me

Sit quietly
Hold my hand
Breathe with me

It's all been said
It's all been done
Let our hearts breathe as one

Know my friend
I will always remain
—in your breath
—in your heart

Breathe with me

• LEY •

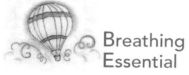

Breathing Essential

Quality of presence is transmitted
through quality of breath.

BLIPP

For those times when you don't know
exactly what to say or what to do,
let your breath convey your caring
(chances are your actions or words
are not what are needed—but your
presence is).

chapter thirty-seven

Breath as a Metaphor for Life

Simplify Down to the Breath

There is much talk these days about the importance of decluttering and simplifying life, whether that be through actions or thoughts. Inspirational author J. J. Goldwag wisely expressed, "There is more to appreciate in every single breath, than in every possession that surrounds you."

For years people told Lynda Austin how important it was to learn to breathe properly. Nevertheless, she just couldn't get into it. As an intuitive life coach, teacher, and workshop leader, she finally felt "I oughta be paying attention." Eventually this awareness led her to a description of the importance of breath. With heartfelt gratitude to Lynda, I share excerpts with her permission.

From Lynda Austin's *Living a Life that Feeds Your Soul: Breath as a Metaphor for Life*

Virtually all of the disciplines will speak to you of breathing, particularly the disciplines that work to simplify life.

Simplify it down to the breath.

Breath, *the breath of life.* Each time you draw in a breath, you create. Each time you breathe out, you present a creation to the world. Each time you breathe in, taking oxygen to your lungs, bloodstream and cells—you become a different human being than you were when you breathed out. You are changed with each breath.

This is life: Experience comes in, experience goes out, and you are changed.

Breath is symbolic in that you cannot take in more than you can use. If you attempt to hold on too tightly, you are *forced* to let go. It is no good to you to try to hold onto it. Think of everything that comes into your life as breath. *He / she / it was a breath of fresh air in my life.* Then why would you want to hold on when it is time to move on, when you know that to hold your breath will kill you?

It is so simple. You cannot take in more than you need, and if you try to hold onto it after you have taken the good out of it, it is of no value to you. You will die. You can only live by letting go, and when you let go, you are then able to take in again.

Consider the person who chooses to give and give and give and is not good at receiving—one cannot breathe that way! You cannot simply breathe OUT. No one blames you if you breathe in. No one says, *Oh, my, isn't she selfish. Look at her breathing up all that air.*

It is so simple. The breath of life. Breath IS life. Life and breath—balanced: in and out. IN is not more important than out. OUT is not better than in.

It is so simple, beautiful, and true. If you learned nothing else in your life, if you would sit and contemplate your breathing, you would understand that such is life.

• • • • •

Ahhhhhhhhhhhhhhhhhhhhhhh There you have it, life simplified down to the breath. As Oprah Winfrey has advised: "What we all want is to be able to live out the truest, highest expression of ourselves as a human being. That doesn't end until you take your last breath."

We are finishing our time together, yet we hope it is the beginning or continuation of a powerful, enriching lifetime journey for you of utilizing the treasure of your breath to thrive.

Dr. George adds:

My Greek grandmother, the under five-foot-tall matriarch on my father's side of the family, was a force to contend with. She presided over a large extended family and was the hub around which our household rotated. When I was a child, we lived right next door, so my sister and I spent considerable time with her. There was little difference in my mind between our house and my grandmother's; they were essentially interchangeable. My sister and I came and went as we pleased.

As much as we were there, every time I left, my grandmother gave me a hug, and in her thick accent told me she loved me, slipped me an olive or two, and gave me a piece of advice: "Be nice to your sister." "Be a good boy." "Pay attention to your parents." "Do what you're supposed to, and come back tomorrow and pull the weeds." I admit that these are not exactly profound pearls of existential wisdom that survive the expanse of space and time; however she sent the message to me that I mattered, that if I set my mind to it, I could positively impact her, my parents, and ultimately my life.

So, like my grandmother, I'd like to leave you with a metaphorical hug and a few pieces of advice.

Perform deep, slow loving breaths and other BLIPPs all throughout your day. Set regular intentions and daily embody one of the attitudes of your choice (beginners mind, non-striving, nonjudgment, patience, trust, letting go, acceptance, kindness, gratitude). Take time to manage your own nervous system, to care for and support yourself and your relationships. Never forget that whether we realize it or not, we impact others through our nervous systems and breath. Be kind, gentle, and loving to yourself, treat yourself to some olives, and don't forget to pull the weeds.

IMAGINE with me please. *It is the future.* By integrating *Breathing Essentials and BLIPPs* into our way of being, together we have made Breath Literacy a "best practice for living" and it has spread around the world.

For the last decades, major universities show substantial research proving benefits of Breath Literacy's Instant Power Practices (BLIPPs): *The breath, in its myriad forms of expression and empowerment, exerts a profound impact on all aspects of health—physical, emotional, psychological and spiritual.* Breath Literacy has been integrated into curricula beginning in preschool and is taught and practiced all the way through graduate studies.

Due to the benefits of Breath Literacy, medications for anxiety, depression, and mental health disorders have significantly decreased. Chronic stress has radically declined. Special "breathing spaces" exist in public areas: waiting rooms, lobbies, airports, schools, etc. "Breathing breaks" are as common as coffee breaks. When many people reach the end of their lives, they have engaged so much breath practice that their last exhale is an easy, natural, letting go.

Preservation of Rainforests, reforestation, and respecting our environment is planetary protocol. We live healthfully longer, and our quality of life is enhanced. There is more love and less violence. For individuals, families, communities, nations, and the world, there is greater well-being. There is greater peace.

"All life breathes together.
Bless each other from the bottom of our heart and soul every day."
• Caroline Myss •

Thank you for taking this journey—this master-course on breath and life! May you feel yourself as an "artist" and a "scientist" and may you continually know blessings in breath moment-by-moment to feed your heart and soul. *Ahhhhhhhhhhhhhhh!*

BREATHE!

With intention
gently
peacefully
gracefully
easily
softly
fully
With purpose
to release
to soften
to ease
to fill
to empty
to loosen
With love
for your body
for your mind
for your spirit
for you
for me
for the world

• Karyn Fulton of BreathLogic •

photo gallery

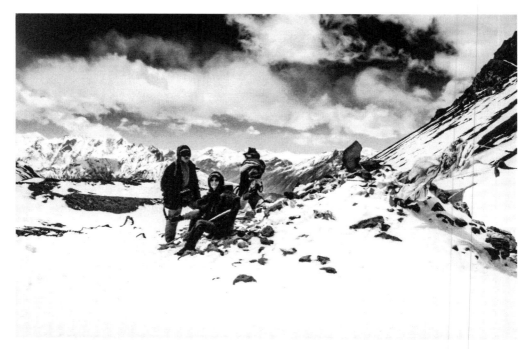

Thorong La Pass, Nepal, 17,769 feet

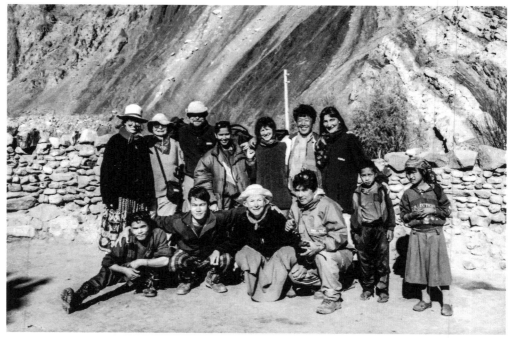

Trekking group (Jason J. Jorgensen)

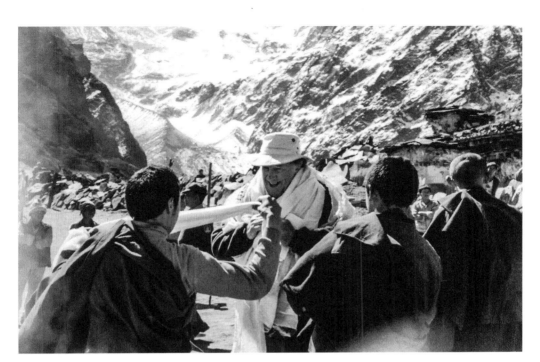

Sir Edmund Hillary, Lukla, Nepal, 40th anniversary

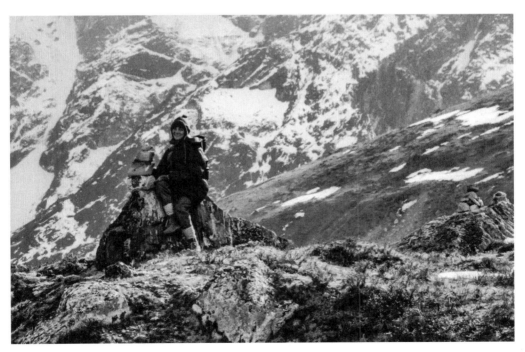

Mountain Majesty at 14,000 feet (Kathleen Fava)

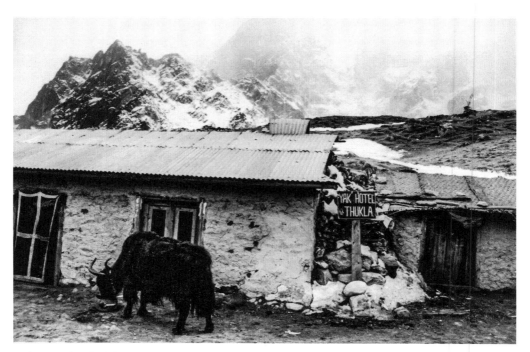

Yak Hotel, Thukla, 15,745 feet

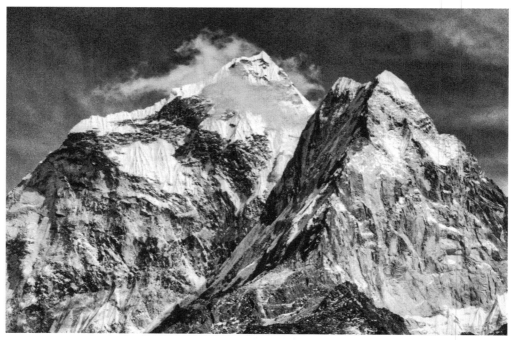

Mount Everest for the Nepalese and Tibetans means "Mother of the Universe"

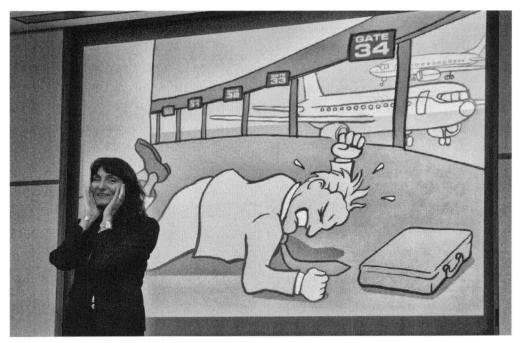

"Tantrum Man" (Nancy Chakrin)

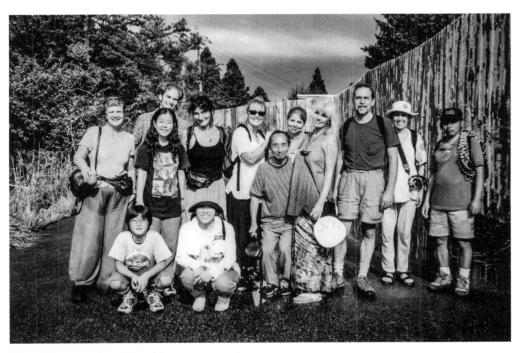

Masaji (center) in Hiroshima (unknown)

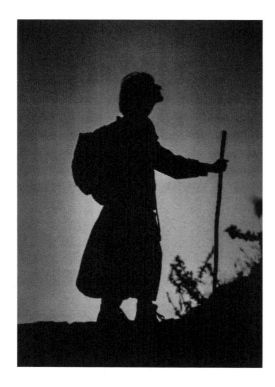

Bip / Bop
Breathing in peace /
Breathing out pain
(Katheen Fava)

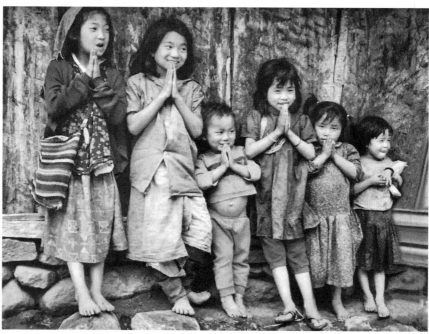

Namaste

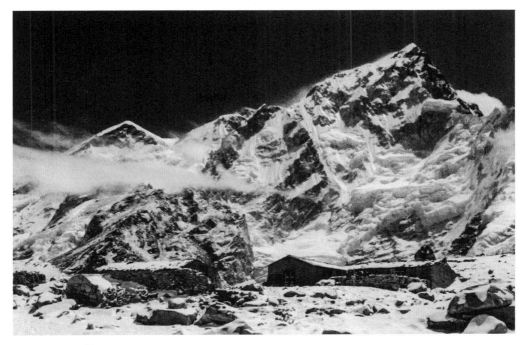

Annapurna Basecamp

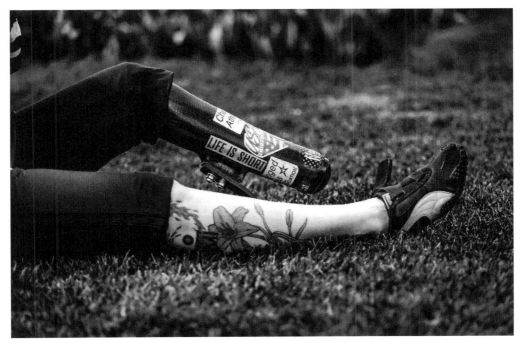

Paralympian Lindsay Nielsen (Ashley Miller)

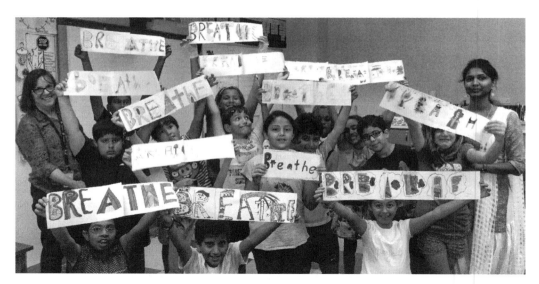

B R E A T H E (George T. Ellis)

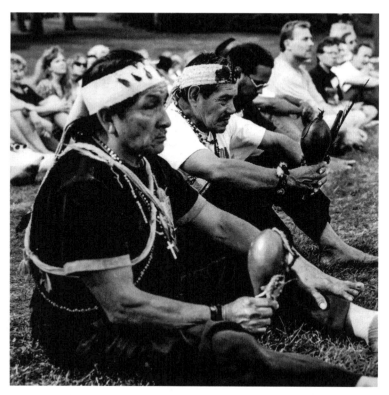

Guarani shamans (Jason J. Jorgensen)

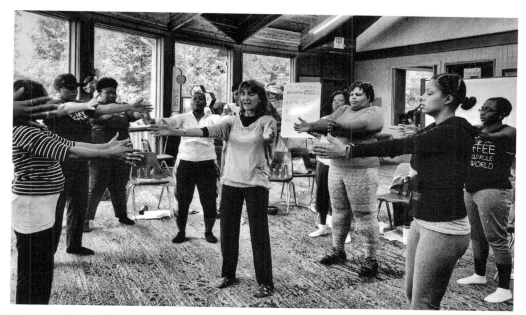

Mentors for Girls Taking Action (Nancy Chakrin)

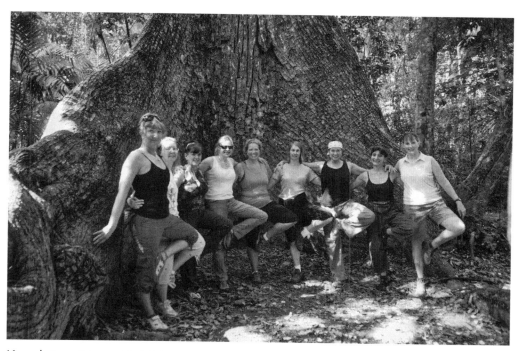

Kapok tree (Nancy Chakrin)

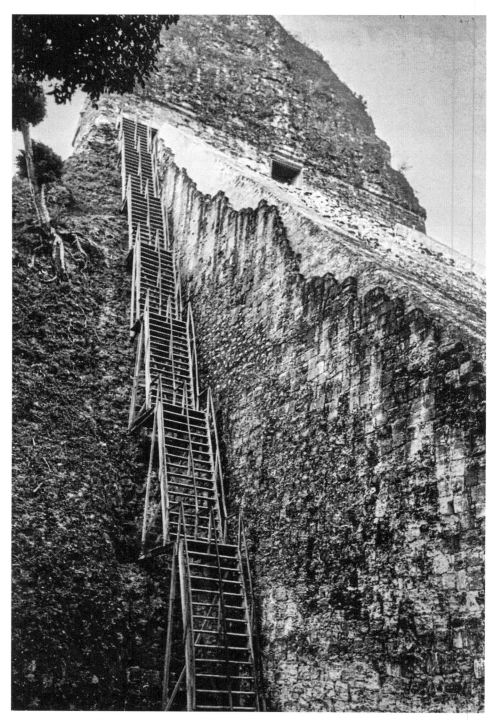

Temple V, Tikal (Richard Britton)

BREATH IS LIFE

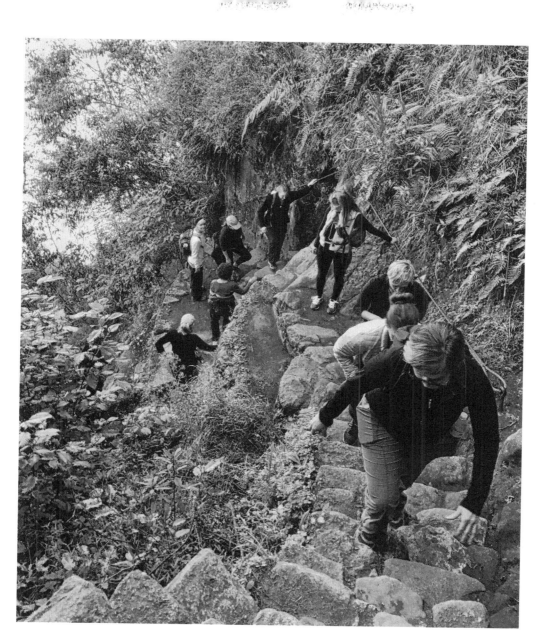

Huayna Picchu, Peru

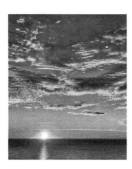

PART ONE: understanding the role of breathing

Each dawn, each inhale—a new beginning
Sunrise from the Costa Blanca, Spain

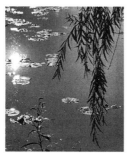

Section I: why breath?

Elements—Forms—Symmetry—Life
Lake of the Isles, Minneapolis, Minnesota

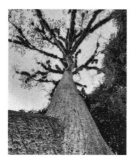

Section II: setting the groundwork

The sky is our limit
Kapok Tree Guardian, Tikal National Park, Guatemala

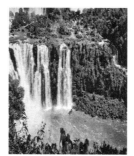

Section III: foundational breathing practices

Exhale—let go . . . Inhale—expand
Iguassu Falls, Brazil

Section IV: your medicine chest

Highlighting healing properties
Rainforests everywhere

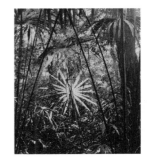

PART TWO: putting understanding into practice

Holding your breath in awe
Majesty of the Andes from Machu Picchu, Peru

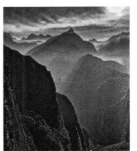

Section V: the right breath at the right time

Volcân Tolimán
Lake Atitlán, in the Guatemalan Highlands

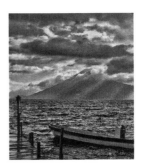

Section VI: breathing throughout life

Each evening, each exhale—a letting go
Sunset on the Red Sea, Arabian Peninsula

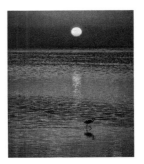

glossary

Ahhhhhhhhhhhhhhhhhhh. *An invitation to savor a long, slow sigh.*

ABC's of Wellness. *Awareness, Balance, Connection.*

Anabolic. *Building up.*

ANS. *Autonomic Nervous System consisting of the SNS and PNS.*

Alternate Nostril Breathing. *A form of pranayama utilizing breathing through alternating nostrils in varying ways for physical and psychological well-being.*

Asanas. *Physical postures of yoga.*

Bandhas / locks. *Concentrated muscular contractions regulating the flow of prana.*

BBH. *"The Brain, the Breath, and the Heart" curriculum.*

Bip / Bop. *Breathe in peace / Breathe out pain.*

BLIPPs. *Breath Literacy's Instant Power Practices that can be accomplished in a "blip" of time or performed for extended periods.*

Breath Geometry. *Geometrical shapes implemented into styles of breathing.*

Breath Literacy. *Knowledge of the art and science of breathing.*

Breathing Ball. *Hoberman Sphere made of hard plastic that expands and contracts.*

Catabolic. *Breaking down.*

EFT. *Emotional Freedom Technique. A form of "energy psychology."*

GTA. *Girls Taking Action. Nonprofit originally called GIA (Girls In Action).*

Glial Cells. *Supportive cells in the central nervous system that surround neurons and provide support for and insulation between them.*

HQ / IQ. *Happiness, Health, Harmony Quotient / Irritation Quotient.*

Hatha yoga. *A yoga system of physical exercises (asanas) and breath control.*

Holotropic. *Breathwork System of psychiatrists Stanislav and Christina Grof.*

Homeostasis. *The state of steady internal physical and chemical conditions creating a dynamic equilibrium for optimal functioning.*

Intuit. *Feel and know at a core level.*

MBSR. *Mindfulness-Based Stress Reduction. An evidence-based training program developed by Jon Kabat-Zinn at the University of Massachusetts Medical Center.*

Mudra. *Sanskrit word meaning "gesture" or "seal." Hand and finger positions believed to aid focus and affect the flow of energy in the body.*

NGO. *Nongovernmental organization, usually nonprofit and humanitarian.*

Neuroception. *Unconscious, ongoing scanning by our brain, for safety and danger.*

Neurons. *Specialized cell transmitting nerve impulses, nerve cells.*

PNS. *Parasympathetic nervous system. Promotes "rest and digest."*

Pausitive. *Being conscious of pausing to notice one's breath, to stop doing to be.*

PG. *Posture and grounding.*

Prana. *Sanskrit word meaning life force contained in the breath.*

Pranayama. *The yogic science of mastering the life force of the breath.*

SBA. *Shallow Breathers Anonymous.*

SNS. *Sympathetic Nervous System. Promotes "fight or flight."*

The 3 N's. *Nurture, Nourish, Nature.*

The 3 S's. *Smile, Soften, Sigh.*

Yoga Nidra. *Known as yogic sleep, a state of deep, conscious relaxation.*

Yogi. *Male practitioner of yoga.*

Yogini. *Female practitioner of yoga.*

Zenulating. *Calming yet energizing at the same time.*

bibliography and resources

Adyashanti. *My Secret Is Silence: Poetry and Sayings of Adyashanti.* Campbell, CA: Open Gate Sangha, 2017.

Allende, Isabelle. "Tales of Passion." [Video] TED Conference, 2007. https://www.ted.com/talks/isabel_allende_tales_of_passion.

Andrews, Bill. "Curing Aging." *Science, Technology & the Future* (Podcast). Feb 25, 2016. https://www.youtube.com/watch?v=sAe5ErMkYMY.

Appeldoorn, Marit E., and Kathy Flaminio. *Moving Mountains: An Integrative Manual to Help Youth with Intensity, Anxiety, and Reactivity.* St. Paul, MN: 1000 Petals LLC, 2020.

Bolen, Jean Shinoda. *Like a Tree: How Trees, Women, and Tree People Can Save the Planet.* San Francisco CA: Conari, 2011.

Bragg, Paul C., and Patricia Bragg. *Super Power Breathing: For Super Energy, High Health & Longevity.* Santa Barbara CA: Bragg Health Sciences, 2008.

Brown, Richard P., and Patricia Gerbarg. *The Healing Power of the Breath: Simple Techniques to Reduce Stress and Anxiety, Enhance Concentration, and Balance Your Emotions.* Boston & London: Shambala, 2012.

Brulé, Dan. *Just Breathe: Mastering Breathwork for Success in Life, Love, Business, and Beyond.* New York, NY: ATRIA, 2017.

Cappy, Peggy. *Yoga for All of Us: A Modified Series of Traditional Poses for Any Age and Ability.* New York, NY: St. Martin's Griffin, 2006.

Carrillo, Maria, Yinying Han, Filippo Migliorati, Ming Liu, and Valeria Gazzola. "Emotional Mirror Neurons in a Rat's Cingulate Cortex." *Current Biology* 29, no. 8 (April 22, 2019).

Charles River Editors. *American Legends: The Life of Jesse Owens.* North Charleston, SC: CreateSpace, 2017.

Cherry, Lynne. *The Great Kapok Tree: A tale of the Amazon Rain Forest.* Orlando, FL: Gulliver Green, 1990.

Chia, Mantak. *The Inner Smile: Increasing Chi Through the Cultivation of Joy.* Rochester VT: Destiny Books, 2008.

Childre, Doc, Howard Martin, Deborah Rozman, and Rollin McCraty. *Heart Intelligence: Connecting with the Intuitive Guidance of the Heart.* Buffalo NY: Waterfront Press, 2016.

Coelho, Paulo. *The Alchemist.* New York, NY: HarperCollins, 1998.

Cook, Diane, and Len Jenshel. *Wise Trees.* New York NY: Publishing, 2017.

Cooper, Bernard. "The Fine Art of Sighing." *The Paris Review.* Summer, 1995.

Corn, Seane. *Revolution of the Soul: Awaken to Love Through Raw Truth, Conscious Healing, and Radical Action.* Boulder CO: Sounds True Inc., 2019.

Cuddy, Amy. "Your Body Language May Shape Who You Are." TED Conference Video. 2012. https://www.ted.com talks/amy_cuddy_your _body_language_may_shape_who_you_are.

Davis, John Francis, Sir. *The Chinese: A General Description of China and Its Inhabitants.* London: Forgotten Books, 2012.

Emmons, MD, Henry. *The Chemistry of Calm: A Powerful, Drug-Free Plan to Quiet Your Fears and Overcome Your Anxiety.* New York, NY: Simon & Schuster, 2010.

Field, Reishad. *Breathe for God's Sake: Discourses on the Mystical Art and Science of Breath.* Xanten, Germany: Chalice, 2013.

Fulford, Robert C. *Dr. Fulford's Touch of Life: The Healing Power of the Natural Life Force.* New York, NY: Pocket Books, 1996.

Fulghum, Robert. *All I Really Need to Know I Learned in Kindergarten: Uncommon Thoughts About Common Things.* New York, NY: Ballantine, 2004.

Gallo, Carmine. *Talk Like TED, The 9 Public-Speaking Secrets of the World's Top Minds.* New York, NY: St. Martin's, 2014.

Gandhi, Arun. *The Gift of Anger: And Other Lessons from My Grandfather Mahatma Gandhi.* New York, NY: Gallery/Jeter, 2017.

Goldberg, Natalie. *Writing Down the Bones: Freeing the Writer Within.* Boulder CO: Shambhala, 2005.

Goldwag, J.J. *Conquering Addiction: A Guide for Maintaining Happiness Regardless of Circumstance.* North Charleston, SC: CreateSpace, 2011.

Goldman, Bruce. "Study shows how slow breathing induces tranquility." Stanford Medicine News Center, 2017. https://med.stanford.edu /news/all-news/2017/03/study-discovers-how-slow-breathing -induces-tranquility.html

Goleman, Daniel. *Destructive Emotions. How Can We Overcome Them? A Scientific Dialogue with the Dalai Lama.* New York, NY: Bantam Dell, 2004.

Goleman, Daniel. *Emotional Intelligence: Why It Can Matter More Than IQ.* New York, NY: Bantam Dell, 2005.

Goodman, John B. *The Road to Self: Reflections from a Soulful CEO*. Chaska, MN: John B. Goodman, 2015.

Goydor, Caroline. "The Surprising Secret to Speaking with Confidence," TEDxBrixton Video, 2014. https://www.youtube.com/watch?v =a2MR5XbJtXU.

Grof, Stanislav, and Christine Grof. *Holotropic Breathwork: A New Approach to Self-Exploration and Therapy*. Albany, NY: State University of New York, 2010.

H.H. Dalai Lama XIV and Howard C. Cutler. *The Art of Happiness. A Handbook for Living*. New York, NY: Riverhead, 1998.

Hallowell, Ed. "6 Reasons Why Mindfulness Begins with the Breath," *Mindful: Healthy Mind Healthy Life,* June 18, 2014. https://www.mindful.org /6-reasons-why-mindfulness-begins-with-the-breath.

Hanson, Rick. *Buddha's Brain: The Practical Neuroscience of Happiness, Love and Wisdom*. Oakland, CA: New Harbinger, 2009.

Hart, Francene. *Sacred Geometry of Nature: Journey On the Path of the Divine*. Rochester, VT: Bear & Company, 2017.

Hawkins, MD, PhD, David R. *Power vs Force: The Hidden Determinants of Human Behavior.* Carlsbad, CA: Hay House, 2002.

Hendricks, Gay. *Conscious Breathing: Breathwork for Health, Stress Release, and Personal Mastery.* New York, NY: Bantam, 1995.

Heriza, Nirmala. *Dr. Yoga. A Complete Program for Discovering the Head-to-Toe Health Benefits of Yoga*. New York, NY: Penguin, 2004.

Hill, Julia Butterfly. *The Legacy of Luna: The Story of a Tree, a Woman and the Struggle to Save the Redwoods*. New York, NY: HarperCollins, 2001.

Iyengar, B.K.S. *Light on Pranayama: The Definitive Guide to the Art of Breathing*. New York, NY: HarperCollins, 2013.

Jacobs-Stewart, Thérèse. *Paths Are Made by Walking: Practical Steps for Attaining Serenity*. New York, NY: Warner Books Inc., 2003.

Jones, Curtis Tyrone. *Guru in the Glass: A Mysterious Encounter While Dying to Live the Unlived Life*. USA: Independently published, 2019.

Kabat-Zinn, Jon. *Full Catastrophe Living: Using the Wisdom of Your Body and Mind to Face Stress, Pain, and Illness*. New York, NY: Dell, 1990.

Kataria, Madan. *Laughter Yoga: Daily Practices for Health and Happiness*. New York, NY: Penguin, 2020.

Kornfield, Jack. *Buddha's Little Instruction Book*. New York, NY: Bantam, 1994.

Kubler-Ross, Elizabeth. *On Death and Dying: What the Dying Have to Teach Doctors, Nurses, Clergy, and Their Families*. New York, NY: Scribner, 2003.

Lauber, Patricia. *Be a Friend to Trees*. New York, NY: HarperCollins and Let's-Read-and-Find-Out Science, 1994.

Lewis, Dennis. *The Tao of Natural Breathing: For Health, Wellbeing, and Inner Growth*. San Francisco: Mountain Wind, 1997.

Lowen, Alexander. *The Language of the Body*. Hinesburg, VT: The Alexander Lowen Foundation, 1958.

MacLean, Paul D. *The Triune Brain in Evolution: Role in Paleocerebral Functions*. New York, NY: Plenum, 1990.

Marvin, Liz. *How To Be More Tree: Essential Life Lessons for Perennial Happiness*. New York, NY: Clarkson Potter, 2019.

Matthiessen, Peter. *Nine-Headed Dragon River: Zen Journals*. Boston: Shambala, 1985.

McAfee, Barbara. *Full Voice: The Art and Practice of Vocal Presence*. Oakland CA: Berrett-Koehler, 2011.

McCabe, Edward. "Viruses and microbes live best in low oxygen environments. They are anaerobic. That means, raise the oxygen environment around them and they die." Mike Garofalo. Benefits of Correct Breathing. *Cloud Hands,* October 8, 2011. http:/mpgtaijiquan.blogspot .com/2011/10/benefits-of-correct-breathing.html?m=1.

McCall, MD, Timothy. *Yoga As Medicine: The Yogic Prescription For Heath and Healing*. New York: NY, Bantam Dell, 2007.

McCarthy, Colman. *I'd Rather Teach Peace*. Maryknoll, NY: Orbis, 2002.

McGilchrist, Iain. *The Master and His Emissary: The Divided Brain and the Making of the Western World*. New Haven and London: Yale University, 2009.

McLuhan, T.C. *Touch The Earth. A Self-Portrait of Indian Existence*. New York, NY: Outerbridge & Dienstfrey, 1972.

Melnychuk, Michael Christopher, Paul M. Dockree, Redmond G. O'Connell, Peter R. Murphy, Joshua H. Balsters, and Ian H. Robertson. "Coupling of respiration and attention via the locus coeruleus: Effects of meditation and pranayama." *Psychophysiology*, 55, No. 9. (September 2018).

Menakem, Resmaa. *My Grandmother's Hands: Racialized Trauma and the Pathway to Mending Our Hearts and Bodies*. Las Vegas Central Recovery, 2017.

Menccagli, Marco and Marco Nieri. *The Secret Therapy of Trees: Harness the Healing Energy of Forest Bathing and Natural Landscapes*. Translated by Jamie Richards. New York, NY: Rodale, 2019.

Merton, Thomas. *Conjectures of a Guilty Bystander*. New York, NY: Doubleday Religion, 2009.

Morningstar, Jim. *The Complete Breath: A Professional Guide to Health and Wellbeing*. Milwaukee, WI: Transformations Incorporated, 2012.

Mushtaq, Romila. "Dr. Romie." *The Powerful Secret of Your Breath*. [Video] TEDx Conference 2014. https:/www.youtube.com/watch?=slKAFdJ8ZHY.

Myss, Caroline. *Invisible Acts of Power: Channeling Grace in Your Everyday Life*. New York, NY: Free Press, 2006.

National Institute of Mental Health (NIMH). "Major Depression." The US Department of Veterans Affairs, VA, 2018. https://www.nimh.nih.gov/health/statistics/major-depression.shtml.

Neff, Kristin and Christopher Germer. *The Oxford Handbook of Compassion Science*. Chapter 27. New York, NY: Oxford, 2017.

Nepo, Mark. *As Far as the Heart Can See*. USA: Freefall, 2020.

Nestor, James. *Breath: The New Science of a Lost Art*. New York, NY: Riverhead, 2020.

Nhat Hanh, Thich. *At Home in the World: Stories and Essential Teachings from a Monk's Life*. Berkeley: Parallax, 2016.

Nhat Hanh, Thich. *Peace is Every Breath: A Practice for Our Busy Lives*. New York, NY: HarperOne, 2011.

Nielsen, Lindsay. Chapter 92 in *Chicken Soup for the Soul: Runners: 101 Inspirational Stories of Energy, Endurance, and Endorphins* by Jack Canfield, Mark Victor Hanson, and Amy Newmark. Cos cob, CT: Chicken Soup for the Soul Publishing, 2010.

O'Dea, James. *Cultivating Peace: Becoming a 21st Century Peace Ambassador*. San Rafael CA: Shift, 2012.

Pakenham, Thomas. *Remarkable Trees of the World*. New York & London: W.W. Norton, 2003.

Porges, Stephen. *The Polyvagal Theory: Neurophysiological Foundations of Emotions, Attachment, Communication, and Self-regulation*. New York, NY: W.W. Norton, 2011.

Price, Verna Cornelia. *The Power of People: Four Kinds of People Who Can Change Your Life.* Minneapolis: JCAMA, 2015.

Rama, Swami, Rudolf Ballentine, and Alan Hymes. *Science of Breath: A Practical Guide.* Honesdale, PA: The Himalayan International Institute of Yoga Science and Philosophy, 1979.

Ramacharaka, Yogi. *Science of Breath.* Chicago, IL: The Yogi Publication Society, 1905.

Rosenberg, Marshall B. *SPEAK PEACE in a World of Conflict: What You Say Next Will Change Your World.* Encinitas, CA: Puddle Dancer Press, 2005.

Selye, Hans. *Stress Without Distress.* Philadelphia & New York: Lippincott Williams & Wilkins, 1974.

Seppälä, Emma M., Jack B. Nitschke, Dana L. Tudorascu, Andrea Hayes, Michael R .Goldstein, Dong T. H. Nguyen, David Perlman, and Richard J. Davidson. "Breathing-Based Meditation Decreases Posttraumatic Stress Disorder Symptoms in U.S. Military Veterans: a Randomized Controlled Longitudinal Study." *Journal of Traumatic Stress,* Aug 27(4):397–405. doi: 10.1002/jts.21936. 2014. 38.

Siegel, Daniel, and Tina Payne Bryson. *The Whole-Brain Child: 12 Revolutionary Strategies to Nurture Your Child's Developing Mind.* New York, NY: Bantam, 2012.

van der Kolk, Bessel. *The Body Keeps the Score: Brain, Mind, and Body in the Healing of Trauma.* New York, NY: Penguin, 2014.

Walker, Matthew. *Why We Sleep: Unlocking the Power of Sleep and Dreams.* New York, NY: Scribner, 2017.

Walker, LCSW, Ruby Jo. Polyvagal Theory: Polyvagal Chart: 2020. https://www.rubyjowalker.com.

Weil, Andrew and Sounds True. *Breathing: The Master Key to Self Healing.* Boulder CO: Sounds True, 1999.

Whyte, David. *Where Many Rivers Meet: Poems.* Langley, WA: Many Rivers, 1990.

Winfrey, Oprah. "Oprah Says She's 'Not Done' Until Her Last Breath." The David Rubinstein Show: Peer to Peer Conversations. March 1, 2017. https://www.bloomberg.com/news]videos/2017-03-01/oprah-says -she's-not-done-until-her-last-breath.

Wohlleben, Peter. *The Hidden Life of Trees.* Vancouver: Greystone, 2020.

World Health Organization. *Newsroom. Fact Sheet Depression,* January 30, 2020. http://www.who.int/news-room/fact-sheets/detail /depression.

Yogananda, Paramahansa. *Autobiography of a Yogi.* The Philosophical Library, 1946.

Zaccaro, Andrea, Andrea Piarulli, Marco Laurino. Erika Garbella, Danilo Menicucci, Bruno Neri, and Angelo Gemignani. "How Breath-Control Can Change Your Life: A Systematic Review on Psycho-Physiological Correlates of Slow Breathing." *National Library of Medicine,* September 2018. https://pubmed.ncbi.nlm.nih.gov/30245619.

acknowledgments

First and foremost I acknowledge George who partners me, breathes with me, and makes me laugh like no one else. Together we honor Bill, Jan, Themeo, and Olga, our parents who witnessed our first breaths as we witnessed their last.

Our most profound thank you to Nancy Chakrin, Marly Cornell, Kate Gregory, Dana Kadue, Melissa Kalal, Dorie McClelland, Mary McDonald, Mary Rains, Pamela Toole, Susan Young, Tim Boyer, Elizabeth Zielenski, and the countless people who contributed directly or indirectly to making this book a reality. We hold all of you—family, friends, publishing experts, advisors, early readers, and BreathLogic board members, past and present—gratefully in our hearts.

I nurture wholehearted gratitude for any yoga, breath, mindfulness, or wellness teachers I have been blessed to study with and who have contributed to my growth and ability to share. I am also deeply grateful to anyone who has ever attended my classes, workshops, retreats, or journeys. In fleeting or memorable ways we connected, enriching each other's stories and lives.

I extend respectful acknowledgment and heartfelt appreciation to every single person whose story we were able to share or whom we mentioned or quoted. May all the narratives, wisdom, and wit touch hearts, inform, and inspire.

Lastly my profound honoring and gratitude for the majesty of this Earth, her mountains, forests/lungs and the air we all share.

Laurie Ellis-Young

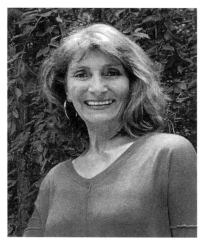

Laurie Ellis-Young MTC, SYT, is an internationally recognized speaker, author, Senior Yoga Teacher (Yoga Alliance U.K.), MBSR instructor, Peace Ambassador (SHIFT), and a pioneer in teaching optimal breathing.

During her early career in the stressful airline industry, Laurie vacationed by leading many adventure-filled treks in the Himalayas and Andes. With limited oxygen, and the highest mountains in the world as her teachers, she discovered the power of breath for "peak" performance, physically and psychologically. She has led groups to over twenty countries including Mexico, Guatemala, Peru, Ecuador, Bolivia, India, Nepal, Thailand, Tibet, Cambodia, France, Spain, and Italy.

Laurie's passion for breath intensified as she sought out various teachers and developed her own personal practice. Desiring to share this knowledge in every way possible, she founded Breathe The Change LLC and cofounded the nonprofit BreathLogic.

George T. Ellis

George T. Ellis PsyD, LP,
is a licensed clinical psychologist with
40+ years of experience in conflict
resolution, stress management, trauma,
cross-cultural psychotherapy, neuropsychology, and MBSR training.

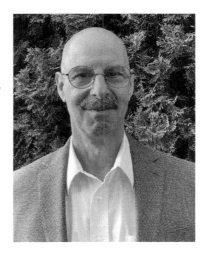

George has been founding director of numerous programs within
global organizations and NGO's
including the UN, USAID, and OSCE
(Organization for Security and Coop-
eration in Europe).

He has practiced as a psychologist and a consultant nationally,
internationally, and privately, in innovative schools, active conflict
zones, telehealth, and the US prison system.

Laurie and George
have lived and worked throughout Latin America, the US, Europe,
Asia, Africa, and the Middle East, experiencing how vital knowledge
of breath can transform and empower individuals, groups, organizations, and systems.

As a way of honoring "trees as the lungs of the planet," for over
twenty years the authors have developed a reforestation project on the
shores of Lake Atitlán, Guatemala.

Please visit BreathLogic.org.

"I'm now BLIPPed for life.

My gratitude to Laurie and Dr. George

for helping me rediscover breathing

as a way of living a full life."

Robert Hetzel PhD
former director of AES
(American Embassy School)
New Delhi, India